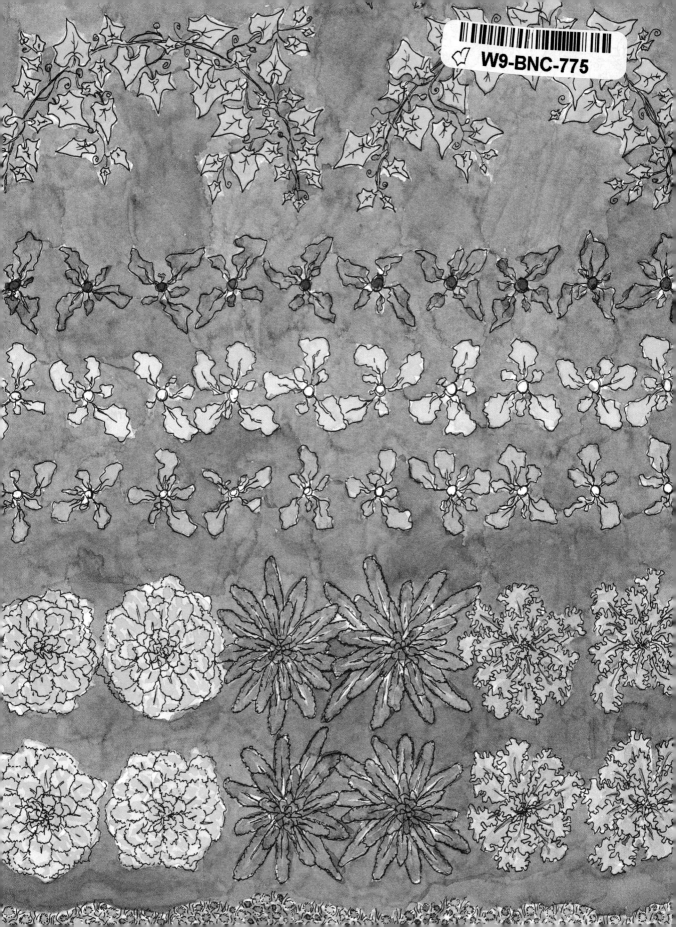

Grow Yourself healthy

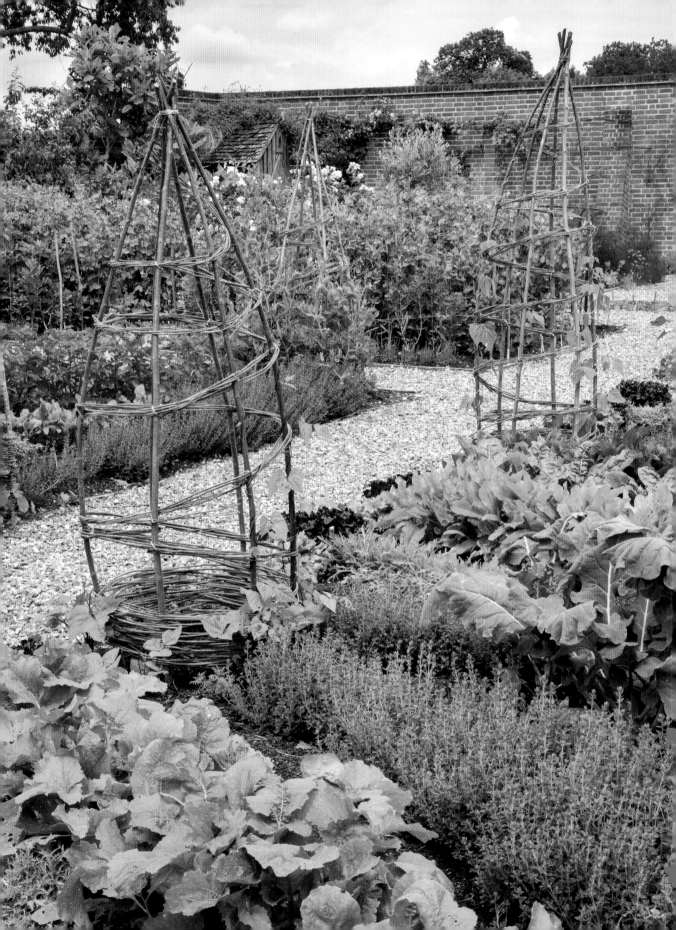

Grow Yourself healthy

Gardening to transform your gut health all year round

Beth Marshall

Photographs by
Marianne Majerus

F FRANCES
LINCOLN

For Annabel

First published in 2020 by Frances Lincoln,
an imprint of The Quarto Group.
The Old Brewery, 6 Blundell Street
London, N7 9BH,
United Kingdom
T (0)20 7700 6700; F (0)20 7700 8066
www.QuartoKnows.com

Text © 2020 Beth Marshall
Images © 2020 Marianne Majerus except where listed on page 191
Copyright © The Quarto Group 2020

A catalogue record for this book is available from the British Library.

ISBN 978 0 7112 5071 0

10 9 8 7 6 5 4 3 2 1

Editorial Director: Helen Griffin
Designer: Rachel Cross
Editor: Zia Allaway
Photography: Marianne Majerus
Illustrator: David Richter
Proofreader: Annelise Evans
Indexer: Michele Moody
Microbiologist: Dr Caroline Le Roy

Printed in Slovenia

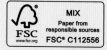

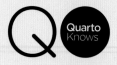

Contents

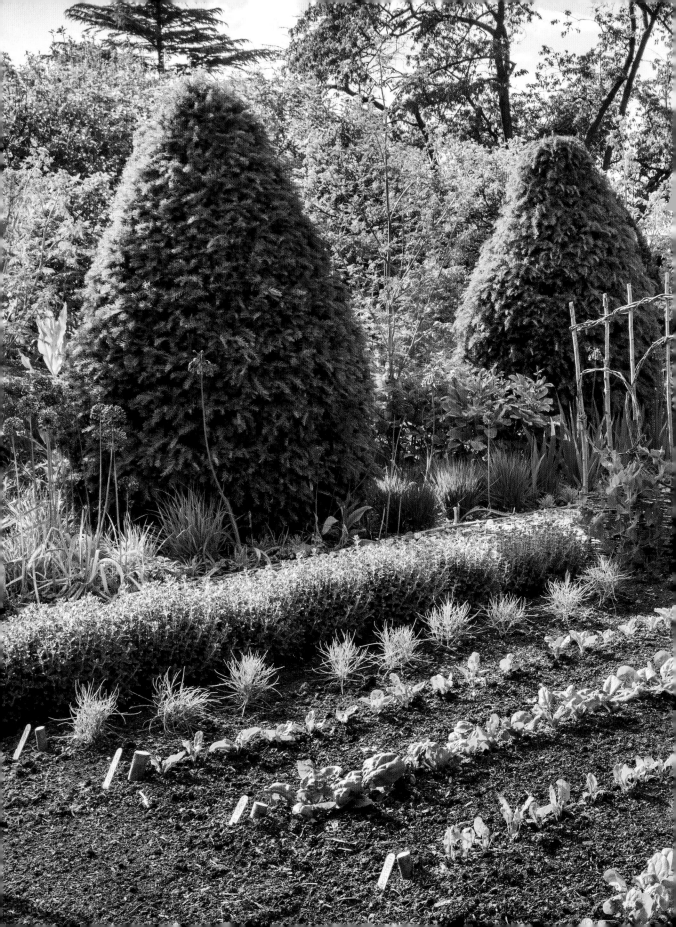

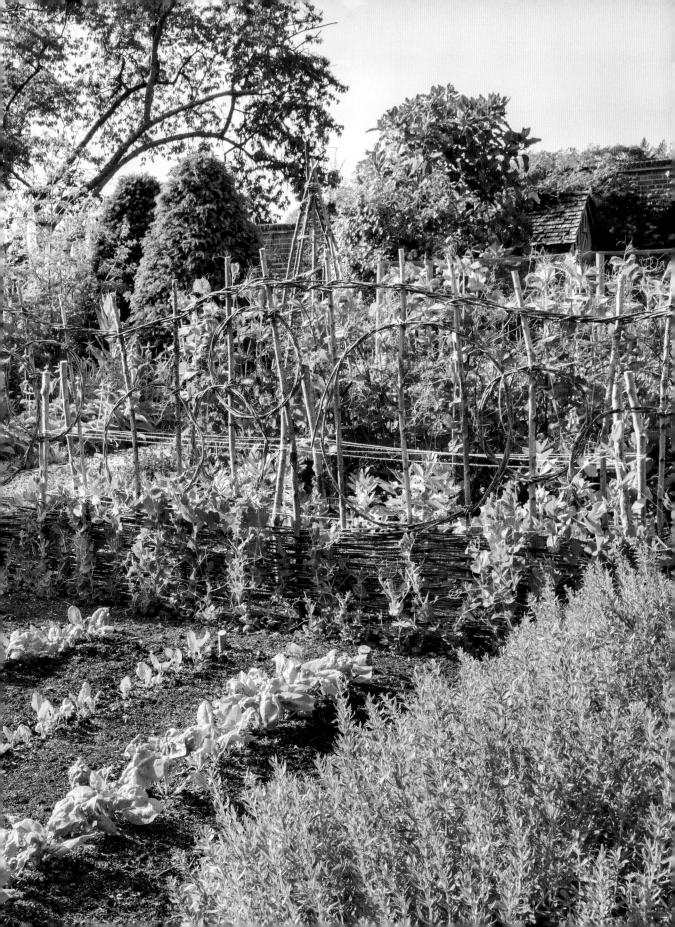

Growing for gut health

Fruit and vegetables provide so many health benefits beyond supplying our basic nutrients. Most people know a punnet of blueberries contains antioxidants that help to protect them from disease, but what's less well known is that the nutritional value of shop-bought berries is a lottery. Their health value will greatly depend on the variety, the conditions the plants have been grown in, and how the berries have been harvested and stored. This same combination of factors applies to almost all types of fruit and vegetable. The good news is that by growing your own crops at home, you can more easily control the health benefits of the foods you eat.

I've looked at hundreds of scientific research papers for this book and described how to grow fruit and vegetables to optimize their nutritional value for you, your family, and the beneficial community of microbes that live within us all, known as the human microbiota. This is the ecosystem of micro-organisms we host within us and interact with in myriad ways. If our relationship with the microbiota breaks down, our health – both physical and mental – can be seriously affected. As a gardener, this is no huge surprise; after all, plants are dependent on an ecosystem of micro-organisms from the soil and the environment in order to survive, so why should we be any different?

Some of the techniques I recommend in this book are contrary to conventional vegetable-growing wisdom. This is partly because the compounds in plants that have the most health benefits accumulate under conditions of stress, such as environmental threats, including exposure to extreme temperatures, nutrient deficiency, drought, or pest and disease attacks. By mimicking these stresses, which plants would experience in more natural conditions, our crops' defences kick into action, and the same compounds that protect them also protect us. Organic techniques can help, too, because plants' defences have to work harder without chemical pesticides, herbicides and fertilizers. Freshly harvested home-grown produce that has not been treated with chemicals or stored for long periods by the supermarkets will also be more abundant in microbial life, which, in turn, can enrich the diversity of our own microbiota.

Aside from using organic methods, there are so many more things we can do to ensure the produce we grow is healthy and nutritious. For instance, home-growers can access a much wider choice of varieties than those on offer in supermarkets. Research shows huge variations between fruit and vegetable varieties, in terms of the health-boosting compounds they contain. Colour is often an excellent indicator of a plant's level of

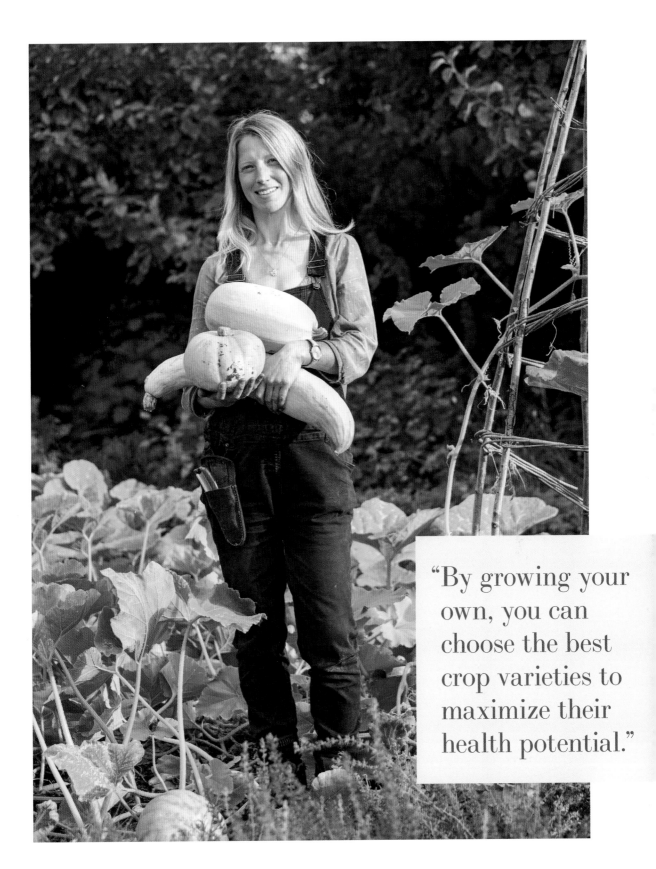

"By growing your own, you can choose the best crop varieties to maximize their health potential."

phytochemicals – compounds that offer powerful defences against disease – while many wild crops and traditional varieties are also rich sources. How we grow, harvest and store our crops also has a major impact on the nutritional value of our food. By buying from the supermarket we have limited control, but if we grow produce at home we can increase the health benefits by ensuring all these conditions are optimal.

A little bit about myself and my motivation for writing this book. Together with my partner, David, I manage the gardens on a 57-acre estate in Berkshire, which includes wildflower meadows, woodlands and ornamental gardens. The beautiful walled garden has a sizeable edible patch and, for someone like me, obsessed with growing wonderful – and occasionally weird – edible plants, planning the vegetable garden is one of my favourite parts of the job. Given the time and effort I put into creating the edible garden, I am keen to make sure there's a scientific reason why growing your own is better than buying from a supermarket. As a professional horticulturist, I have always been interested in growing nutritious food, but after starting my family – I have two children under the age of three – I want to ensure my little ones are weaned on the healthiest, plant-based diet.

The other principle to remember is that because everyone's microbiota is unique, diversity in your edible garden is the key to good gut health. The different compounds in the plants that we eat interact with each other in ways that are only just starting to be understood. Growing a broad range of fruit, vegetables, herbs and nuts to eat offers the best way to nurture your beneficial microbes, rather than eating processed foods or taking supplements.

I have also included the world of fermenting in these pages. Most people will already be consuming fermented foods, such as cheese, yoghurt, olives and wine, but if you've not tried making your own fermented fruits and vegetables before, you'll be amazed by the taste and nutritional benefits. Try my simple recipes to transform the produce you've lovingly grown into foods that will benefit your microbiota, or experiment with flavours to create your own fermented treats.

In researching and writing this book, this book I am very grateful for the assistance of Dr Caroline Le Roy, Research Associate at King's College London, for reviewing the scientific aspects of my research to check that it's all factually correct, and suggesting additional interesting references. Thank you so much for sharing my enthusiasm about the concept of this book and being so generous with your time and support.

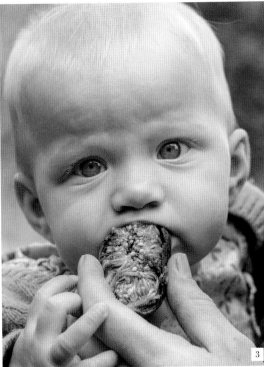

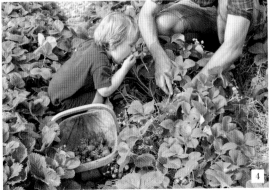

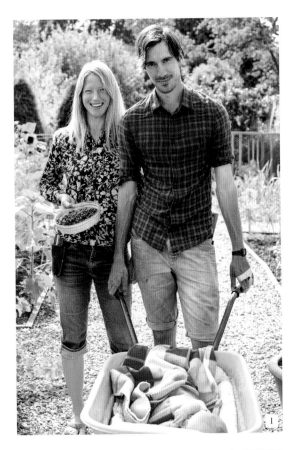

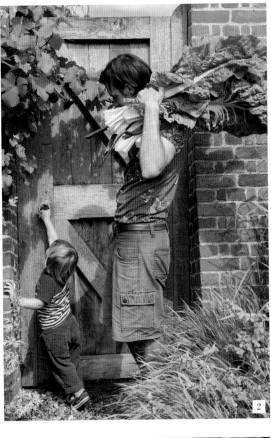

1. *Beth and David in the garden with baby Fern.* **2.** *Frank helps David harvest a crop of nutritious Swiss chard.* **3.** *Weaning babies on a wide range of fruits and vegetables helps them to establish a rich and diverse microbiota.* **4.** *Strawberries are easy to grow and make a perfect snack for children.*

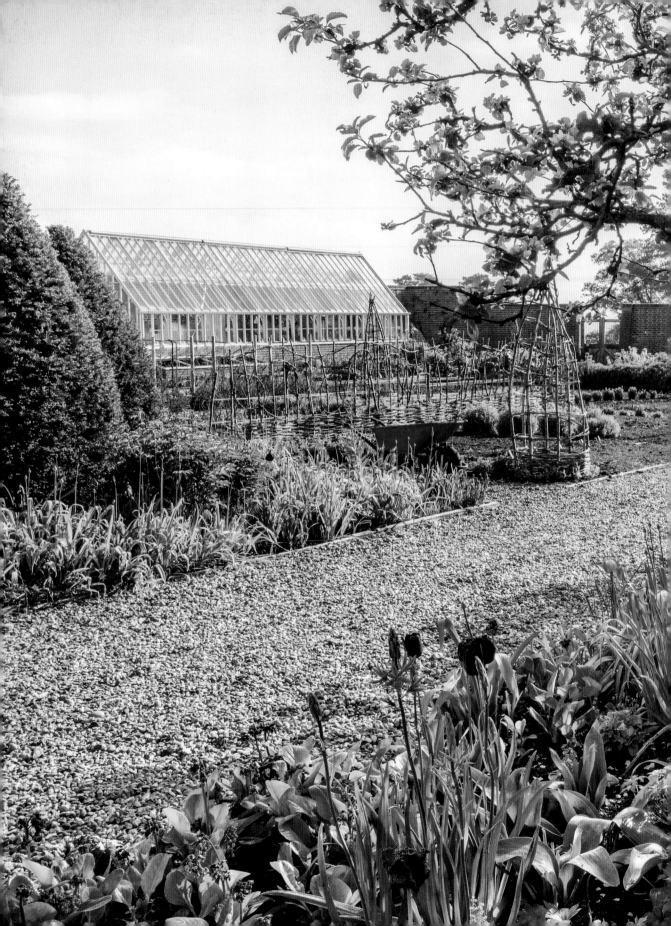

CHAPTER ONE

The Science Explained

"Understanding the relationships between humans, plants and microbes is the key to unlocking good health and wellbeing."

Why focus on gut health?

Nourishing the trillions of beneficial microbes that live in our gut helps us to fight disease and ward off mental illness, and the key to keeping them in peak condition is in the food we eat.

Recent research shows that there is more than a little truth to the old adage, 'you are what you eat'. Studies have linked gut health to our physical and mental wellbeing and there is a wealth of evidence that shows how eating a plant-based diet plays a crucial role in ensuring that we host a healthy, diverse community of microbes.

Humans are inhabited by trillions of microbes living within and on us. The collective mass of our microbes is called the microbiota, which contains over a thousand different known species of organism. In fact, on average we are only about 43 per cent human; the remaining 57 per cent is made up of microbes that work like an additional organ. Critical to maintaining the healthy functioning of the human body, each person's microbiota is different and unique, like a biodynamic fingerprint.

The gut microbiota helps us to digest our food and unlocks nutrients our bodies would otherwise be unable to access. Amazingly, over 70 per cent of our immune system is also found in the gut, which explains why eating a plant-based diet that boosts our microbiota also helps to protect us against diseases and disorders.

Microbes play a key role in manufacturing vitamins and regulating cholesterol, and they help to protect us against heart disease and cancer, as well as warding off diabetes by improving insulin resistance. In addition, they have a positive effect on our mental health by creating compounds, such as serotonin, that influence brain function, memory and reasoning.

The composition of our microbiota is determined by a myriad of factors, which include our genetic make-up, where we are from, how we were born, if we were breastfed, whether we have taken antibiotics, our sleep patterns, age, stress levels, and, very importantly, our diet. Recent science shows how commonplace illnesses, such as diabetes and obesity, Alzheimer's disease, allergies, and anxiety and depression, could be due to a breakdown in the relationship we have with our microbiota.

CHANGING DIETS

Our relationship with our microbes has evolved over millennia, but modern eating patterns have changed rapidly, shifting from a diet rich in unprocessed plant wholefoods packed with dietary fibre, to one high in animal fats, animal proteins, refined sugar and highly processed products.

The food we eat not only nourishes us but also has an impact on the composition of our inner microbial ecosystem. While we may not all be lucky enough to inherit a robust gut microbiota, the dietary choices we make have a significant effect on it. Much of the food essential for these beneficial microbes, such as fermentable fibre (see pages 16–19), comes exclusively from plants, and research increasingly shows that they hold the keys to good health.

Right *Eating a varied and diverse diet of organic home-grown produce does not just provide us with nutrient-packed goodness, it also nourishes our ecosystem of microbes for better gut health.*

"Eating a plant-rich diet feeds our gut microbes, which help to improve our physical and mental wellbeing."

Food for our microbiota

Plants contain a number of important compounds that benefit our gut microbes. Fibre in its many forms is particularly good for health and the fruit and vegetables you grow at home offer an abundant source.

To design an edible garden with gut health in mind, we first need to understand what makes plants so beneficial to our microbes. They contain essential nutritional components that help our digestion to work efficiently and feed our gut microbiota (see page 14), which protects us from many diseases and disorders of both the body and the mind.

HOW PREBIOTICS WORK

Compounds in plants that benefit our microbes are often referred to as 'prebiotics'. They work like fertilizers for our microbes, stimulating the growth and diversity of beneficial bacteria in our gut. The most important prebiotics in plants are different types of carbohydrate, including resistant starch and fructans, which our microbes break down and ferment to produce health-enhancing beneficial compounds, such as short-chain fatty acids (SCFAs).

SCFAs help to regulate a healthy digestive system, increasing the acidity of the gut, which reduces the growth of harmful bacteria. They also help to maintain a strong mucous layer, making the gut less permeable and preventing inflammatory problems, such as inflammatory bowel disease (IBD). Prebiotics boost numbers of 'good' bacteria in the gut, improving nutrient absorption and increasing SCFA production. In addition, they help to protect against Type 2 diabetes and heart disease, while stimulating the growth of immune cells in the gut.

Prebiotics are found in other substances, too, such as human breast milk. As well as nourishing babies, breast milk contains oligosaccharides, which we are unable to digest. They pass into the gut where they fuel babies' microbes and promote a healthy digestive system. Honey also contains oligosaccharides, and experts now consider it to be prebiotic.

FOOD FOR MICROBES

All plants are rich in dietary fibre, the tough material we find difficult to digest. Fibre-rich foods cannot be digested in our small intestine and pass through into the large intestine (colon), where some is broken down and fermented by our microbes, producing SCFAs. Other types of fibre are not fermented, or at least only slowly, but are still beneficial, absorbing water and bulking up our stools to help speed up our bowel movements. We are all advised to eat 30g/1oz of fibre per day but few of us manage anywhere near as much. A nutritional survey showed that to meet this daily dose, men need to increase their fibre intake by 50 per cent, and women by an incredible 75 per cent.

STARCH FACTS

Plants store energy as starch, a complex carbohydrate that they break down into glucose, which they use for growth or development. While we can digest glucose, some starch in plants is made of tougher stuff that resists being digested, just like fibre. It too passes through the small intestine into the large intestine, where microbes convert it into beneficial compounds, such as SCFAs. Good sources of resistant starch include wholegrains and seeds, such as bread, oats, cereals, pasta and rice; potatoes; firm bananas; peas and beans; squashes; and sweet potatoes. These filling plant foods also ward off

HOW PLANTS FEED OUR GUT MICROBES

This chart shows how the food we eat is either digested in the small intestine or passes through into the large intestine, where it is broken down by microbes.

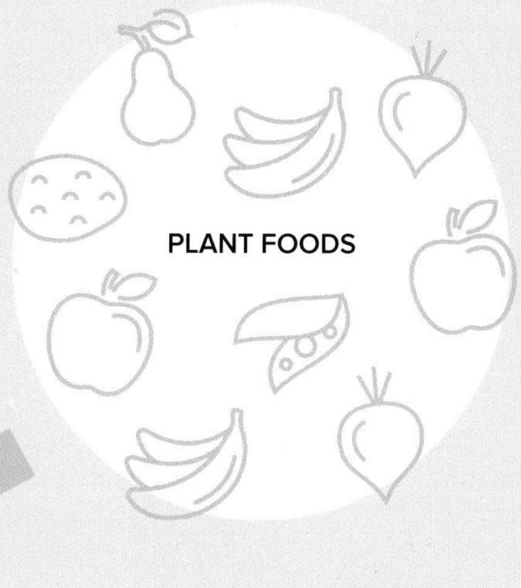

Eating plant foods
Whole fruits, vegetables, herbs, nuts and wholegrains contain macronutrients, such as protein, fat and carbohydrates, including fibre and starch, as well as vitamins and minerals. Plant foods also contain health-promoting phytochemicals.

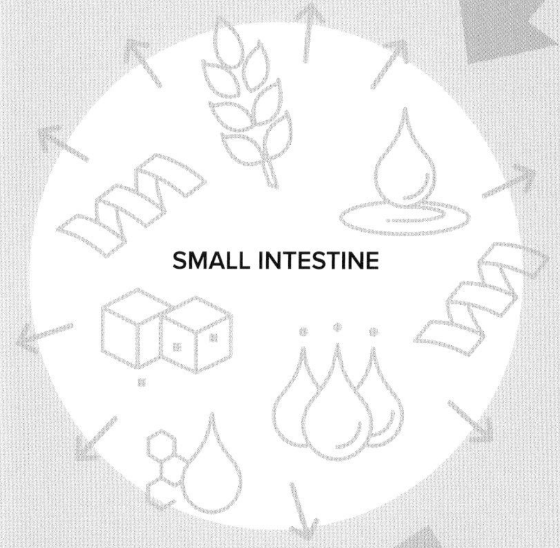

PLANT FOODS

Our food is firstly broken down mechanically by chewing in the mouth and pounding in the stomach, before it passes into the intestines for digestion.

SMALL INTESTINE

Digestion in the small intestine
90–95 per cent of the food we eat is broken down and absorbed into the body in the small intestine. Most macro- and micronutrients are easily absorbed, but fibre and starch resist digestion.

Indigestible dietary fibre, including resistant starch and fructans, and phytochemicals pass from the small to the large intestine.

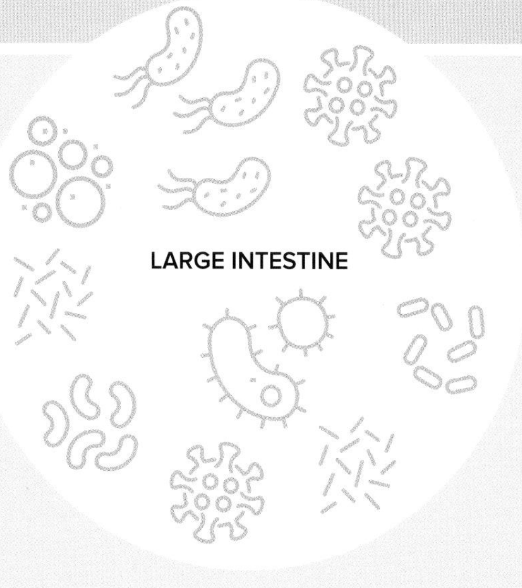

Digestion by microbes in the large intestine
Most microbes reside in the large intestine and help us to absorb nutrients by breaking down dietary fibre, phytochemicals and some vitamins. Microbes produce short-chain fatty acids and other molecules that help to increase our immunity and support good physical and mental health. The large intestine also helps to absorb fluids and process waste.

LARGE INTESTINE

ESSENTIAL VITAMINS AND MINERALS

Minerals and vitamins are known as micronutrients and are essential to our health, even though the body uses them in small amounts. We also need tiny quantities of trace nutrients, such as iron, manganese, zinc and selenium. Many of these nutrients are found in a range of plant foods.

VITAMIN	FUNCTION	EXAMPLES OF FOOD SOURCES
Vitamin A	Important for healthy eyesight and organ functioning.	Vegetables rich in carotenoids, such as carrots, squash, sweet potatoes, spinach, liver, dairy products, fish.
B vitamins	Help the body convert carbohydrates into energy; produce red blood cells and lower cholesterol. They also assist in brain functioning.	Peas, beans, nuts, seeds, wholegrains, dark green leafy vegetables, asparagus, citrus fruit, avocados, bananas, eggs, dairy products, meat.
Vitamin C	Essential for the growth and repair of tissues in the body. Helps in the development and functioning of the nervous system. Required for the production of collagen, which is needed for healthy skin.	Cabbages, kale, Brussels sprouts, dark green leafy vegetables, citrus fruit, tomatoes, squash, peppers, potatoes.
Vitamin D	Essential for a healthy immune system. It also assists with the absorption of calcium, enabling healthy bone development.	Fatty fish (such as salmon), some dairy products, egg yolks. Our bodies also make vitamin D from sunlight on our skin.
Vitamin E	Acts as an antioxidant. Helps establish a strong immune system and is important in the formation of red blood cells.	Seeds (such as sunflower), nuts (almonds, hazelnuts, peanuts), dark green leafy vegetables, vegetable oils, such as corn, sunflower and soybean.
Vitamin K	Needed in blood clotting, it also helps to ensure healthy bone development.	Dark green leafy vegetables, winter squash, liver, cheese, legumes such as peas and beans.
MINERAL		
Calcium	Needed for bone and teeth formation. Helps the functioning of blood vessels and muscles.	Dairy products, leafy green vegetables (especially brassicas), peas, beans, nuts.
Phosphorus	Essential for the formation of healthy bones and teeth, and helps the body to store energy.	Dairy products, nuts, seeds, peas, beans, wholegrains.
Magnesium	Involved in many bodily processes, including muscle and nerve functioning, regulating blood pressure, and protein and bone synthesis.	Green vegetables, fruit (kiwi, figs, some berries and bananas), wholegrains, nuts, seeds, peas, beans, artichokes, avocados, asparagus, fatty fish.
Sodium	Helps to balance water levels in the body, regulating blood flow.	Salt, meat, cheese, beetroot, spinach, Swiss chard, celery, artichokes.
Chloride	Works with sodium to help balance fluids and blood flow in the body.	Seaweed, salt, lettuces, celery, tomatoes, olives.
Potassium	Helps to maintain blood pressure, regulates muscle contractions and ensures the nerves function properly.	Bananas, citrus fruit, legumes, melons, apricots, some dried fruit, cooked spinach, squash.
Sulphur	Present in every living tissue in the body. It is an important building block in the development of proteins.	Garlic, onions, leeks, chives, cabbages, kale, Brussels sprouts, asparagus.

hunger for long periods, therefore eating them can help to reduce obesity.

FRUCTANS FOR HEALTH

Some flowering plants conserve energy in the form of a particular type of fibre called fructans, rather than starch. Fructans enable plants to tolerate stressful conditions, such as drought or extreme temperatures. There are a few different types, such as inulin and fructooligosaccharides (FOS), that contain valuable prebiotic fibre for our microbes.

• **Fructooligosaccharides** have a sweet, mild taste and are sometimes used to sweeten processed foods. They are fermented by gut bacteria more quickly than inulin.

• **Inulin** has a savoury taste and fatty, velvety texture. It takes longer to ferment and produces SCFAs, mainly in the form of butyrate, that strengthen the lining of the gut, reducing the risk of inflammation. Several studies show important links between butyrate, the nervous system and brain function, referred to as the gut-brain axis.

The form of fructans is not always constant, and levels may vary according to different environmental conditions, such as temperature shifts and availability of water. This means that the fructans most dominant in a plant may differ according to the way it is grown and when it is harvested. Fructans-rich crops include Jerusalem artichokes, asparagus, chicory roots, peas, beans, and globe artichokes, as well as unusual types, such as dandelions (see also the Vegetables & Fruit in Focus chapter on pages 38–121).

CHEMICAL ATTRACTION

As well as dietary fibre, plants contain other compounds known as phytochemicals, which have health-promoting properties beyond those provided by vitamins and minerals. Recent studies show phytochemicals lower the risks of cancer, heart disease, diabetes, inflammation and age-related eye disease. Many act as antioxidants, protecting cells in the body from damage caused by free radicals. As most phytochemicals are not absorbed in the

small intestine, our gut microbes help us to break them down, increasing the numbers and diversity of beneficial bacteria in the process. More beneficial bacteria means an increase in the production of health-boosting compounds, such as SCFAs.

All plants contain a complex mix of phytochemicals, which have multiple effects on human health. There are thousands of different types, including polyphenols, which are particularly good for our microbes and our health. These chemicals are a plant's defence system. Conditions of stress, such as extreme heat, ultraviolet (UV) rays, and the threat of attack from pests and diseases, trigger a surge of them in a plant. Phytochemicals also play a role in attracting beneficial insects and birds by dictating flower colour, taste and scent. In addition, they help to prevent infections in a plant and regulate its growth.

Without phytochemicals we wouldn't be able to enjoy the rich sensory experience of eating food, since they also determine a plant's flavour. Some may impart a bitter taste – think of the slight acridity of chicory and mustard, or the tannins in tea – which is logical from the plant's point of view, since they are designed to protect it from harm, including being eaten by us.

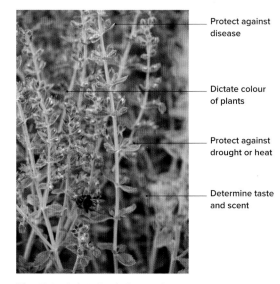

Protect against disease

Dictate colour of plants

Protect against drought or heat

Determine taste and scent

The effects of phytochemicals on a plant such as Teucrium.

Grow a rainbow

To maximize the nutritional benefits of the food we grow, it's essential to select a rainbow of fruit and vegetables that provide many different types of phytochemicals and a feast for our gut microbes.

Colour is an excellent indicator of the health value of fruit and vegetables – brightly coloured plants contain different types of phytochemicals that offer a range of health-boosting properties. Here are a few groups of phytochemicals that are especially beneficial for our gut health and wellbeing.

POLYPHENOLS

These are present in lots of brightly coloured foods and are the most abundant source of antioxidants in our diet. They help to protect us against various different types of cancer, cardiovascular disease, allergies and inflammatory health issues. Polyphenols include flavonoids, such as anthocyanins, which are present in many red and purple foods. Other flavonoids include capsaicinoids (in chilli peppers); resveratrol (in red wine); ellagic acid (in berries); and lignans (in seeds).

CAROTENOIDS

Found in many orange, yellow and red foods, such as carrots, tomatoes and squash, carotenoids have anti-cancer properties and help to protect against cardiovascular diseases and degenerative eye disease, while also strengthening the immune system. Carotenoids include phytochemicals called lycopene and carotenes, which break down in the body where they are converted to vitamin A (see page 18).

SULPHUR COMPOUNDS

Cruciferous vegetables, such as kale, broccoli, and Brussels sprouts, contain sulphur compounds called glucosinolates. Alliin is another sulphur compound found in members of the onion family, including garlic, leeks, onions and chives. These compounds tend to give the plants their bitter taste, or their pungent smell when you chop or cook with them, and are very beneficial to health, reducing the risk of cancer and protecting the heart and immune systems.

By growing a diverse range of fruit and vegetables from the five different colour groups – purple/blue, red, yellow/orange, green and white – we can help to maximize the levels of different types of phytochemicals we eat in our diet.

Why grow white?

Although white vegetables are not bright and rainbow coloured, many are excellent sources of beneficial phytochemicals. Onions, garlic, cauliflower, potatoes, parsnips, daikon radishes, celeriac and mushrooms, for example, all contain important phytochemicals, including alliin, quercetin, and sulforaphane, which help to prevent cancer, increase bone strength, lower cholesterol and reduce inflammation.

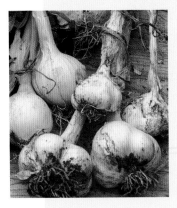

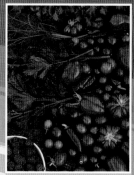

Red

Crops to grow
Tomatoes, red peppers, red onions, beetroot, berries.

Health benefits
Helps to prevent cancer, especially prostate cancer; reduces the risk of heart disease and stroke.

Phytochemicals
lycopene, anthocyanins, ellagic acid

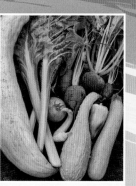

Orange/yellow

Crops to grow
Carrots, squash, golden beetroot, sweetcorn, yellow peppers, sweet potatoes, citrus fruit, such as oranges, pineapples, melons, peaches.

Health benefits
Promotes healthy vision and cell growth in the skin; increases blood circulation; lowers the risk of cardiovascular diseases.

Phytochemicals
carotenoids, lutein, zeaxanthin, hesperidin

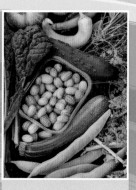

Green

Crops to grow
Broccoli, kale, Brussels sprouts, spinach, Swiss chard, green beans, peas, courgettes, asparagus, green apples, green grapes.

Health benefits
Improves blood and bone health; enhances the immune system; helps to prevent cancer.

Phytochemicals
glucosinolates, lutein, zeaxanthin

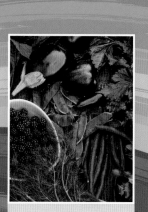

Purple/blue

Crops to grow
Berries, aubergines, plums, figs, grapes, purple cultivars of vegetables, such as kale, potatoes, onions, broccoli, and lettuce.

Health benefits
Helps prevent cancer, oxidative stress and inflammation, and protects cells from damage.

Phytochemicals
anthocyanins, resveratrol

Aim for diversity

Leading nutritionists recommend that we eat at least 30 different types of fruits and vegetables a week, and this can be easily achieved by nurturing your own diverse organic garden of culinary delights.

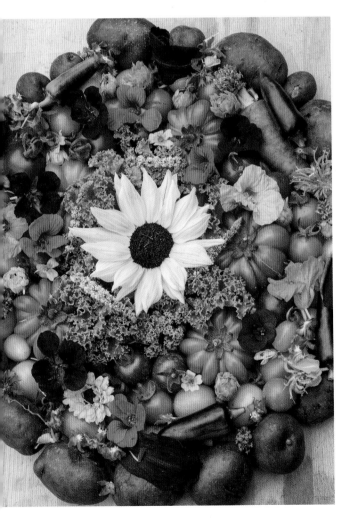

Increasing diversity in our diet not only benefits us nutritionally, it can also enliven our palette with colours, tastes and scents.

"Low diversity of gut microbes has been shown to increase the risk of bowel disease, diabetes and arthritis."

We all need to get more diversity into our diets. Currently, over half of our energy needs comes from just five crops – rice, wheat, maize, millet and sorghum. These grains are often highly processed in food products, which decreases their nutritional value further. Not only does this limit diversity in our diets, compromising our own health and that of our microbes, it also compromises the health of our global ecosystems.

Vast tracts of natural habitats are cleared to make way for farming, eroding the ecosystem services they provide and threatening wildlife. This type of mass food production also makes the land and crops very vulnerable to threats such as drought, flooding, and pest and disease outbreaks, which are all exacerbated by global climate change. We can help to reverse this worrying trend by growing as diverse a range of edible plants as possible, which will also contribute to maintaining genetic diversity, increasing biodiversity and creating sustainable food production.

The human gut microbiota is like an ecosystem (see pages 16–19). The diversity of species living within us, and the number of microbes within those species, will dictate the resilience of our immune system. Think of it in terms of the vegetable garden – if you grow a few different varieties of bean and one is particularly susceptible to blackfly, at least you have others to harvest. Diversity is critical for our health, too, as studies show a link between low microbial diversity in the gut and inflammatory bowel syndrome, arthritis, Type 1 and 2 diabetes, Crohn's disease and obesity.

Different bacteria consume different types of 'fuel', so to create a diverse ecosystem in the gut it is important to provide them with as many different types of fruit, vegetables and herbs as possible. Scientific understanding of which foods benefit our microbiota is evolving, but focusing on a limited number of food types, such as those recommended in restricted diet plans, is likely to exclude a whole range that would be beneficial to our gut microbes.

Dieticians recommend that we aim to eat at least 30 different types of plant a week. Try to get up to 50 if you can, by including small quantities of plants, such as herbs and spices, that are high in polyphenols. Also vary the types of plants you eat over the course of a month and a year by growing seasonal produce.

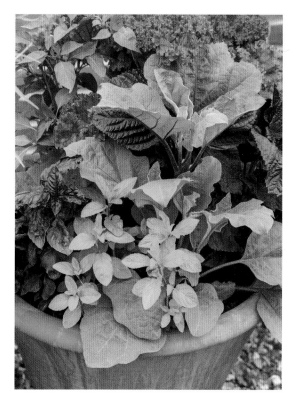

We do not necessarily need a large garden to grow for diversity if we make use of smaller spaces with productive pots, such as this container filled with a range of herbs and vegetables.

BROADEN YOUR RANGE

The joy of growing your own is that you can select from a vast range of vegetables, fruit, herbs and seeds, which are more interesting than the limited number of varieties available in supermarkets. The fresh produce we can buy in the shops also tends to be the easiest to grow commercially, focusing on yield or storage potential rather than flavour, which is also important to our microbiota.

The only limit to the diversity you can grow is how much space and time you have. However, even in a small garden or on a balcony you can grow a wide range of crops, especially if you select dwarf varieties. Check out the Grow-for-health Projects chapter for ideas: I have created containers and small raised beds filled with different crops for you to try (see pages 124–27; 136–39; 144–49).

I focus on growing small quantities of a wide range of produce, planting one crop after another in succession to make the most of the space, and preventing large gluts that we can't eat or store. In our garden, we grow over 150 varieties of annual vegetables, in addition to a wide array of fruit bushes and trees, herbs and perennial crops. Foraging among them for relatively small quantities of food to add to multi-ingredient meals is fun and appeals to a broad range of hungry gut microbes.

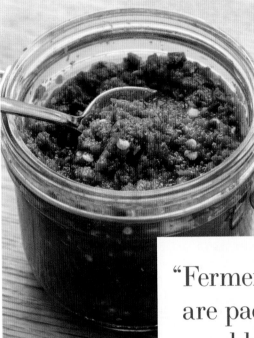

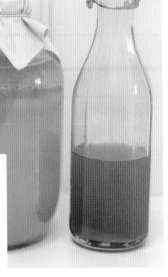

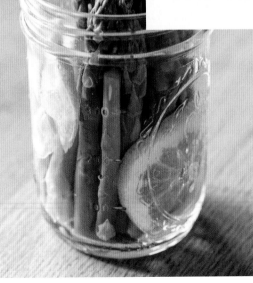

"Fermented foods
are packed with
good bacteria
that help increase
our immunity
to diseases."

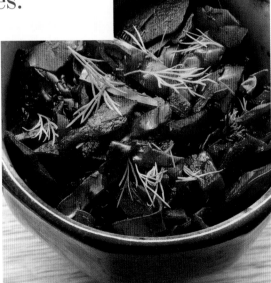

Secrets of ferments

Fermented fruit and vegetables, such as pickles and sauerkraut, are known as probiotics and are extremely good for our gut health. They're also easy to make and a great way to store home-grown crops.

Transforming your home-grown fruit and vegetables into probiotics is another great way to enhance your health. Probiotic foods contain live cultures of bacterial micro-organisms, such as *Bifidobacterium* and *Lactobacillus*, and when these are eaten in the right quantities, they can increase the diversity and numbers of beneficial bacteria in the gut.

Probiotics can be made by fermenting the edibles we grow in our garden to produce a whole array of delicious pickles, kraut, kimchi, and flavoured fermented drinks, such as kombucha and kefir (see pages 164–81 for recipe ideas).

PROBIOTIC ALCHEMY

Probiotics can help to support a healthy digestive system, guarding against intestinal disorders, such as irritable bowel syndrome (IBS), abdominal pain and bloating. They also support a healthy immune system, working to prevent allergies or problems associated with inflammation. Research shows they offer benefits to mental health, the reproductive system, oral health, skin and the respiratory system. Fermentation increases acidity, too, which protects the preserved foods from being colonized by harmful bacteria.

Although probiotics have many benefits for our health, guaranteeing precise results can be difficult because it is impossible to determine exactly which strains of bacteria are present in fermented produce, and in what quantities. It's also difficult to tell how many of those strains will go on to implant populations of microbes in the gut. Think of it a bit like guerrilla gardening and throwing seed bombs into a field. A few seeds grow on to establish healthy plants, but many will not germinate. Injecting microbial populations into the gut is similar. However, if we eat fermented foods regularly enough and over a long period, our gut microbiota is more likely to be diversified and improved, along with our health.

PHYTOCHEMICAL INCREASES

Another amazing fact I have discovered is that the process of fermentation also increases the amount of phytochemicals, such as polyphenols and flavonoids, in food (see pages 20–21). This is because, as fermentation occurs, the plants' cell walls are broken down and phytochemicals are released, making them available for our bodies to absorb.

The process of fermentation also affects the degree to which polyphenols and flavonoids are increased, which means the health benefits of your foods will vary depending on the length of time they are fermented for, the temperature they are stored at, and other environmental factors.

Why not experiment with fermented foods and see for yourself? For me, they have been an absolute revelation. The transformative genius of microbes to make fermented produce offers a fun and creative way to store and use your home-grown crops.

Clockwise from top left *Fiery chilli ferment; rhubarb kombucha, a delicious drink made from fermented tea; sauerkraut made with red cabbage; pickled asparagus tips with lemon.*

The plant microbiota

Just as we have a microbiota made up of microbes that defend us against diseases and ailments, so do plants, and we can benefit from theirs simply by eating a diet rich in organic fruit and vegetables.

Plants are supported by a community of microbes, just like us, and we can help to ensure this microbiota is enriched and nurtured. Research into the plant microbiota is in its infancy, but studies are unravelling the critical role it plays in supporting a plant's growth and protecting it against disease.

New research is also looking at how human and plant microbiotas may be interconnected. Studies show that eating some types of organically grown raw fruit and vegetables may provide an important source of microbes that could colonize the human gut, increasing our own microbial diversity. One study of apples found the flesh and core, in particular, are excellent sources of beneficial bacteria. Just picked, organically grown apples also have a more diverse bacterial community than conventionally grown crops, and these bacteria can even help to enhance the flavour of the fruit (see also pages 104–107).

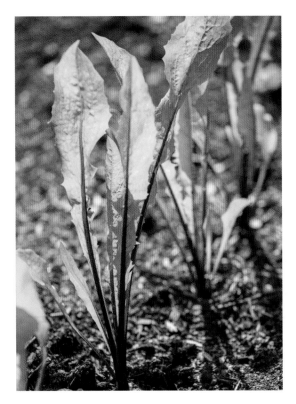

HOW PLANTS' MICROBES EVOLVE

A plant's microbiota is passed on from its parents via the seed. Amazingly, the microbiota in wild plants can also be affected by microbes passing from the guts of birds and animals that eat and distribute the seed.

The microbes of germinating seeds and seedlings are affected by many external factors, including the soil's acidity and organic matter, water availability, and other environmental conditions. Wild plants have evolved with microbiota specific to their habitats, but, as a result of plant breeding and modern cultivation techniques, this relationship has been disrupted, leading to a significant degradation of the plant microbiota and to disease outbreaks. Synthetic inoculants of bacteria are being developed to address this problem, with mixed results, but using organic techniques, which protect the health of plant microbes, is a far more sustainable long-term solution.

Left *Organically grown produce has a more diverse and balanced bacterial community than conventionally grown crops, making them better for our health and enhancing their flavour.*

Five ways to enrich the plant microbiota

Research into plant microbiotas has found the greatest abundance and diversity on farms that limit soil disturbance, minimize the use of fertilizers, and protect biodiversity – all growing methods we can adopt at home. Try these easy ways to protect your plants' microbes and maximize the benefits to you in the process.

1. Grow organically and avoid the use of chemical pesticides, herbicides and fertilizers These types of pesticides, herbicides and fertilizers can have a detrimental impact on the communities of microbes in plants and in the root zone. Follow organic practices and avoid using chemicals to optimize the health of the plant microbiota in your garden.

2. Save your own seed Plant microbiotas are passed on from one generation to the next via the seed. Some seed companies use chemical pesticides and herbicides that may have a detrimental impact on the plant microbiota, limiting the microbial diversity that's passed on to the seeds. Furthermore, some companies clean and treat their seed during processing in ways that also harm plant microbiotas. By saving our own seed, or buying it from sources we know use organic practices, we will help safeguard the relationship between the plant and its microbes.

3. Use 'no-dig' growing systems Minimizing soil disturbance by not digging the soil can also help to minimize the disruption to root-associated microbial communities. A no-dig system simply means leaving the soil undisturbed and planting or sowing directly into it, rather than digging it over every year.

4. Include organic matter Making your own compost, or sourcing organic types, such as manure, mushroom compost or composted

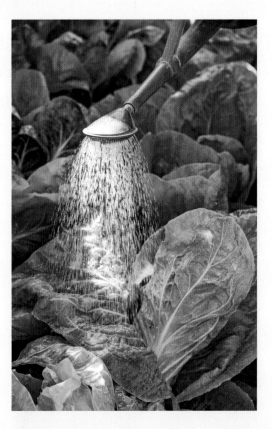

green waste, and spreading it over the surface in a thick layer – known as a mulch – improves the soil structure, increases its nutrient- and water-holding capacity and provides an excellent environment for microbial and fungal populations in and around the plant roots. Mulch your beds with a layer of organic matter 5–7cm/2–3in deep annually and worms and micro-organisms will incorporate it into the soil naturally.

5. Add your own microbial populations Douse the soil with compost teas or plant ferments (pictured above) to increase the diversity of microbes. Find out how to make these nutrient-rich ferments on pages 150–51.

Stress is best

There are a few tricks to growing healthier crops and most will surprise seasoned gardeners because they are contrary to the conventional wisdom that experts have been recommending for many years.

As gardeners, we all have a tendency to mollycoddle our crops and give them the optimum conditions for growth, but new research shows that this can actually reduce their health benefits. This is because phytochemicals (see pages 19–21), with their health-boosting properties, often accumulate in plants that are stressed. Growing plants for their nutritional value requires quite a radical shift in the way we think, but we have to remember that plants wouldn't be here today if they could not adapt to adversity. Phytochemicals provide plants with a natural defence system, protecting them from detrimental changes to the environmental conditions around them. They're like chemical warfare against pest damage and strengthen the plant's ability to cope with difficult growing conditions, such as drought or prolonged heat, cold, or intense sunlight.

It follows that if we create conditions where plants are out of their comfort zone, they should then increase their phytochemical content. For example, we can expose them to greater UV levels by planting them in full sun, or grow them outside rather than under cover to increase temperature differences between day and night, or decrease the amount of fertilizer we use. Avoiding pesticides can also help to increase phytochemicals. Plant varieties with natural resistance to pests and diseases, usually marketed as 'disease resistant', often contain higher levels of these beneficial compounds. Obviously we don't want to stress plants so much that yields are significantly affected, but we can find a balance to optimize the nutritional value of the food we grow.

FLUCTUATING PHYTOCHEMICAL LEVELS

How long crops are left to mature also has a definite impact on their nutritional value. Different types and levels of phytochemicals are present in a plant at different stages of its development. Key stages when shifts happen are when seeds germinate, as the leaves develop, at the point of flowering, and when the plant produces fruits and seeds.

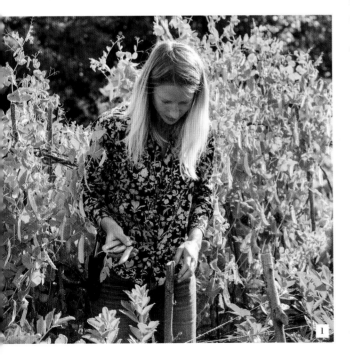

1. Don't worry if you spot a few pests as they will encourage your plants to accumulate more beneficial phytochemicals. **2.** *Growing crops outside in cold temperatures can boost phytochemical levels.*

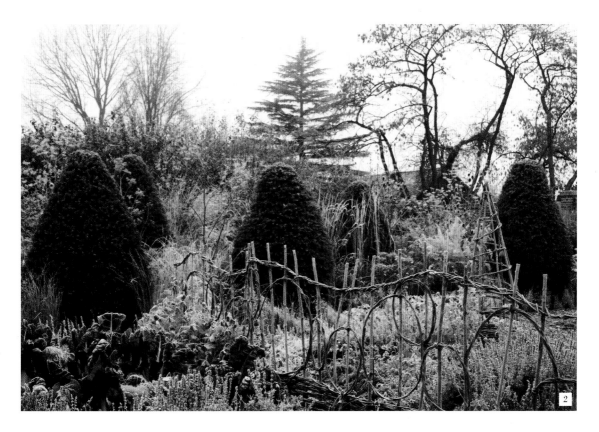

2

"Some fertilizers, such as nitrogen, have an adverse effect on plants' phytochemicals."

For example, when a seed germinates, a massive surge in phytochemical levels helps to protect the seedling from the environmental threats it faces as it enters the world, such as intense sunlight or extreme temperatures. Polyphenols in mung beans, for instance, increase by an incredible 2,010 per cent

from dormant seeds to seven-day-old seedlings. Levels of polyphenols, which give plants their flavours, are very high in leaves during their early stages of growth, helping to protect them from being eaten or damaged. As a plant is about to flower, polyphenols accumulate in the blooms, creating colourful pigments and scents to attract pollinators, and when seeds start to develop different types of phytochemical form to protect them from decay.

Fruits reaching maturity use phytochemicals to attract animals and insects that disperse their seed. For example, some berries have bright red and purple colours due to a type of phytochemical called anthocyanins. So, picking the fruit when it is ripe and colourful should maximize its phytochemical levels. Having some knowledge of how and why these compounds develop in the plant can really help us as gardeners. We can then make sure we're harvesting our produce at the best possible stage of growth for the most health benefits.

Choosing what to grow

Growing your own fruit and vegetables introduces you to a whole range of healthy crops, and opting for wild species and traditional, local varieties will afford even greater nutritional benefits for home-growers.

"95 per cent of the world's food energy needs comes from just 30 different types of plant."

Although the way we grow edible plants can drastically affect their nutritional values, the genetic make-up of fruit and vegetable varieties is probably the most significant factor in determining their nutritional profiles. Every different variety, or cultivar (a plant bred for a specific quality not found in its natural form), of crop has a unique genetic code that dictates the level of nutrients and phytochemicals it contains. There can be a huge variation, especially in terms of phytochemicals, even within an individual type of crop. For example, a study into hundreds of different varieties of potato found some cultivars contained 15 times more phytochemicals than others. Some also contain a much greater diversity of different types of phytochemical. Therefore, by growing a range of different varieties we can increase the diversity of the food we eat. This will then provide different types of fuel for different strains of microbe in our guts, which will promote better health.

There are hundreds of varieties of crops available, often selected to suit the local growing conditions in different regions of the world, offering a huge array of genetic diversity – far greater than the choices offered for sale at the supermarket. As gardeners we can tap into this world of diverse nutritional benefits by growing different, unusual varieties from seed.

The types of produce at the supermarket are often also selected for their high yields or uniformity of look, rather than their nutritional value. In addition, plant breeders in recent years have tended to select varieties with milder, sweeter flavours for the consumer, but these are not necessarily the best for our health. For example, some people find the taste of Brussels sprouts bitter, so breeders have selectively grown plants with a milder taste profile. The original bitter flavour is due to a key compound called glucosinolates, which has many benefits, such as improved cardiovascular health and protection against cancer. Growers have increasingly selected plant food varieties that may have lower levels of phytochemicals, reducing the potential health benefits they provide.

SELECTING FOR NUTRITIONAL VALUE

While I would love to give you a shopping list of the best varieties to choose for their nutritional value, information on the phytochemical content of foods is only available for some of the named varieties of fruit and vegetables you can grow. These are often crops that are available only locally in specific parts of the world, which makes recommendations of specific varieties tricky. In this book, I've focused mainly on

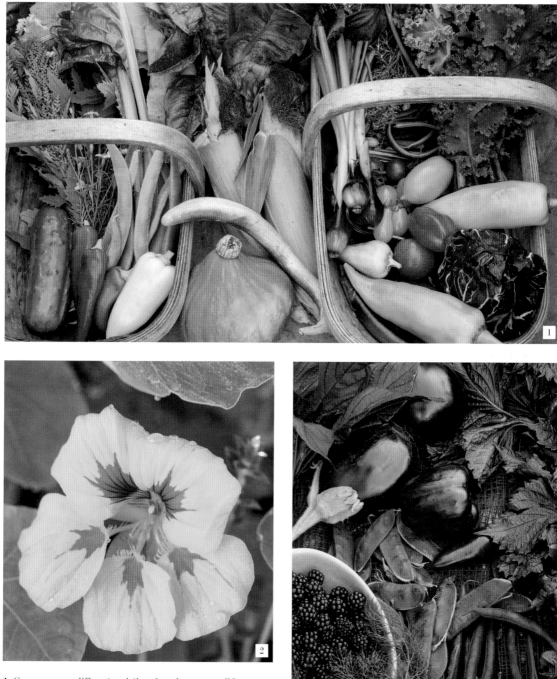

1. *Grow as many different varieties of produce as possible, as plants with different genetic profiles have different phytochemical contents.* 2. *Edible flowers, such as nasturtiums, are often high in polyphenols.* 3. *Strong colours, such as these purple crops, are often an indicator of a crop's high nutritional value.*

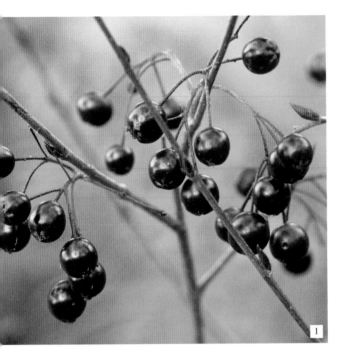

crop varieties with specific features that are linked to their nutritional value. For example, colour is often a strong indicator of phytochemical content, and brightly coloured fruit and vegetables often have high levels of polyphenols. Please note, however, that this is not always true, as some pale-coloured crops, such as onions and garlic, also contain highly beneficial phytochemicals (see pages 20–21).

The size and shape of a crop can also be useful in helping us to choose healthy varieties – small fruits, for example, often have higher levels of phytochemicals than larger fruits.

For the future, an aspirational vision for the horticultural industry would be for seed catalogues to rate cultivars of fruit and vegetables based on nutritional value and to provide growing advice to optimize their benefits to health.

GROWING WILD

In many cases, wild food crops have higher levels of phytochemicals and antioxidant activity than cultivated varieties. This is partly because over the years growers have selected and bred varieties that have lower nutritional value, favouring for example larger fruits, or less bitter flavours with lower levels of phytochemicals, and consequently antioxidant activity. For example, wild blueberries have two or three times the level of polyphenols of cultivated varieties. Similarly, studies show that wild blackberries have four to five times more polyphenols than cultivated types. Berries from naturally occurring plant species, such as elderberries and chokeberries, have been ranked consistently at the top of charts of edible plants with the highest polyphenol content. It is likely that these fruit and vegetables are more nutritious because of their genetic make-up, and also because of the more stressful environmental conditions they experience during their lifetime.

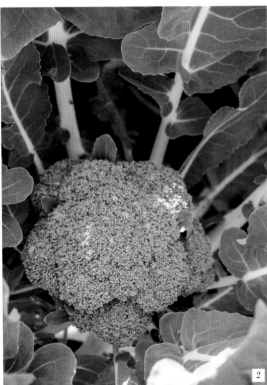

1. Chokeberries (Aronia) have been found to have the highest polyphenol content of any berry. 2. The chemicals that give brassicas, such as broccoli and Brussels sprouts, their bitter flavour also protect humans from harmful bacteria and disease.

KEEPING UP WITH TRADITION

In many cases, local, traditional cultivated varieties, sometimes called 'heritage' varieties or 'landraces', also contain higher levels of polyphenols and antioxidant activity. This is likely to be because, like their wild counterparts, traditional varieties have had to survive in more stressful environmental conditions and develop defence mechanisms in the form of phytochemicals. For example, there are hundreds, if not thousands, of traditional apple-tree varieties, and many studies have shown they contain a much richer treasure trove of polyphenols than modern cultivated types. These traditional apple trees may not yield such high numbers of crops, but make up for it in health benefits, not to mention more interesting flavours and textures than supermarket-bought fruit.

We can tap into these phytochemical-rich edibles in a number of ways. Firstly, we can find and grow local, traditional varieties. Not only are they more healthy, but sourcing them is also an interesting way to find out about your local agricultural heritage. Secondly, we can grow naturally occurring species of edible plants, and mimic natural conditions by subjecting them to a degree of stress.

Many nurseries will stock some types of native wild plants you can easily grow in the garden, such as blackberries or elderberries. Other naturally occurring species may not be as easy to source, but you can often grow plants from seed as an alternative.

The Food and Agriculture Organization of the United Nations (FAO) estimates that there are about 100,000 different under-utilized species of edible wild food plants we could be including in our diets. At present 95 per cent of the world's food energy needs comes from just 30 different types of plant, so why not be adventurous and select some more unusual food plants to grow in your garden? It makes sense to increase your dietary diversity and also to support more genetic diversity in our food systems.

Lastly, we can forage from the wild – reliving the experiences that our parents enjoyed – while making sure we don't pick endangered or toxic species.

Wholefoods for health

From the point of view of your gut microbes, growing your own fruit, vegetables, herbs, seeds, nuts and, in an ideal world, grains, is preferable to eating highly processed foods for a number of good reasons:

- **The plant cells** of wholefoods are more likely to reach the large intestine intact, providing more fuel for your beneficial microbes and increasing gut health.
- **Food additives**, including artificial sweeteners, often used in processed foods, have a negative effect on the beneficial bacteria in your gut.
- **Different components** of wholefoods, such as phytochemicals, fibre and nutrients, interact in complex ways that are not yet fully understood. These interactions may be essential to the ways in which plant compounds are broken down and absorbed by the body.

Currently, it is impossible to tell from food labelling the extent to which wholefoods are present in processed products. However, by growing and eating your own organic food you can be confident you're providing yourself and your microbes with 100 per cent plant-based goodness.

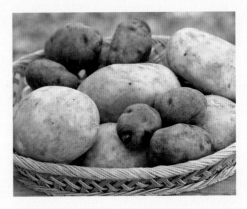

Dispelling myths

Most of us assume that fresh food is better for us than produce that has been stored or cooked, and that organic crops have the highest nutrient levels, but scientific studies reveal a different story.

There are a number of widely held beliefs about which foods are the most nutritious and the best ways of growing and storing them that recent research is now questioning. For example, most of us would assume that freshly harvested fruits and vegetables are better for us than those that have been put into storage, but that is not always the case.

ORGANIC FOODS ARE MORE NUTRITIOUS?

As an organic grower, I would really like to say with confidence that organic food is better for you and your gut microbiota, but so far the scientific evidence is mixed. Although there are many environmental benefits to organic methods of growing food and to the plants' microbiotas (see pages 26–27), there is currently no clear proof to back up the claim that organic food is better in terms of basic nutrition.

In the last two decades two scientific reviews that looked at hundreds of trials comparing organic and conventional growing methods could not find clinically significant differences in basic nutrient levels, with the exception of phosphorus, which is found in greater quantities in organically grown crops. However, even phosphorus is not present in levels that are 'clinically significant', and it is also not needed in high quantities to sustain human health – we would need to be almost starving to show symptoms of phosphorus deficiency.

Similarly, although levels of pesticide residues are higher in people consuming conventional rather than organic produce, they are not at levels deemed to be a health risk. Still, the use of environmental pollutants, such as chemical pesticides, fertilizers and herbicides, do have an adverse effect on the microbiotas of plants and humans, potentially also negatively affecting our health in turn.

While organic food may not be better in terms of basic nutrition, organically grown crops contain significantly higher levels of phytochemicals (see pages 19–21), according to a scientific review. The scientists calculated that a switch to organic produce would increase the polyphenols by 20 to 40 per cent. So why is this the case? The reason seems to be because phytochemicals, and antioxidants, increase when plants are grown under conditions of stress – crops grown organically are likely to be at greater risk from pest and disease attack, or more stressed due to a lack of fertilization. Crops grown without the use of pesticides are likely to have richer and more diverse plant microbiota too. An important recent French study also showed that people who regularly eat organic food are less likely to develop cancer.

VEGAN DIETS ARE HEALTHIEST?

Most people would assume that because vegan diets are totally plant-based and high in dietary fibre they would be better for the gut microbiota. Vegan diets also tend to be higher in folic acid, vitamins C and E, minerals such as potassium and magnesium, and, of course, many phytochemicals. A logical assumption

Right *Organically grown crops have a more diverse microbiota and higher phytochemical content that benefit our health. Eating organic food has also been linked to a reduced cancer risk.*

"Many crops accumulate more health-promoting phytochemicals when stored for a while."

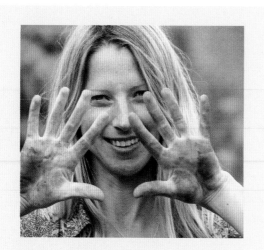

Dirt causes disease?

The very act of gardening and getting your hands dirty helps to increase the diversity of your microbiota. Gardening is a great way to 'meet' more microbes; a single teaspoon of garden soil can contain up to one billion bacteria. Bacteria are highly adaptable, and studies into mice show that exposure to soil microbes increases microbial diversity in the gut. Increased bacterial diversity is linked to a reduced risk of certain diseases. Our ancestors had close contact with the soil but modern lifestyles are increasingly disconnected from nature, leaving us out of touch with the world of microbes around us.

Modern agricultural techniques that use chemicals and the sterilization of many processed foods also mean the crops we buy are often very depleted in microbial life from the soil. However, as gardeners we can address this imbalance. If we ensure we manage our soil well, nurturing biodiversity and getting our hands dirty enough, our health can benefit from these rich microbial ecosystems. It's also another great reason not to peel your fruit and vegetables.

is that more plants equals more fibre, equals a more diverse and resilient microbiota. However, while it's true that plant-based diets foster the development of a more diverse gut microbiota when compared to those of omnivores (people who eat meat and plant foods), studies so far indicate there is little difference between the microbiota of people following vegan or vegetarian diets. Vegan diets also have other challenges. Certain dietary components, such as protein, iron and vitamin B-12 are more difficult to access when eating an entirely vegan diet and some careful planning is needed to ensure people include a wide enough variety of fruits, vegetables (including pulses) and wholegrains for their nutritional needs. These findings reinforce the central message of this book: eat a plant-based diet that is as diverse as possible for a healthy, resilient microbiota.

Plant-based diets, high in fibre and phytochemicals, also lead to an increase in the numbers of beneficial bacteria, such as lactic acid bacteria, in the gut, compared to the microbes found in the digestive systems of those who eat meat. More beneficial bacteria lead to an increase in the production of short-chain fatty acids (SCFAs), which play such an important role in health and wellbeing (see pages 16–19). Plant-based diets are also better for the environment, causing less pressure on natural ecosystems and fewer greenhouse-gas emissions.

GLUTEN-FREE IS GOOD FOR THE GUT?

So, what other factors influence the composition of the gut microbiota? Gluten-free diets for one. Studies into people on gluten-free diets show that most have lower numbers of key beneficial microbes, and an increased risk of heart disease. Low FODMAP (Fermentable Oligosaccharides, Disaccharides, Monosaccharides and Polyols) diets are also currently very popular. These restrict the intake of carbohydrates, such as fructans, lactose and fructose, and have been found to reduce the symptoms of irritable bowel syndrome (IBS). However, because they restrict excellent sources of fuel for gut bacteria they can also have a negative impact on the gut microbiota. Consequently, it is best to consult a healthcare expert before following one of these diets.

Fresh is best?

Eating fresh produce is not necessarily better for our health, especially when we look at the phytochemical content in plants. Before I started this research, I assumed eating crops as quickly as possible after harvesting would be better nutritionally. To my surprise, most fruits and vegetables seem to accumulate more beneficial phytochemicals while in storage, although they may lose fructans and vitamins (see pages 16–19). Beneficial microbes in fresh produce may also deplete over time. However, drying has an impact, often increasing phytochemical levels. For example, dried herbs usually have significantly higher levels of polyphenols than fresh.

Many raw foods are not best either. For example, we are able to absorb the lycopene in tomatoes much more easily if they are cooked. Other types of phytochemicals in carrots and asparagus are also more accessible when the foods are heated.

1. Cook tomatoes to increase the levels of lycopene that the body is able to absorb. *2. The polyphenol content of some crops, such as carrots, increases while they are in storage.* *3. Levels of resistant starch increase in stored sweetcorn.*

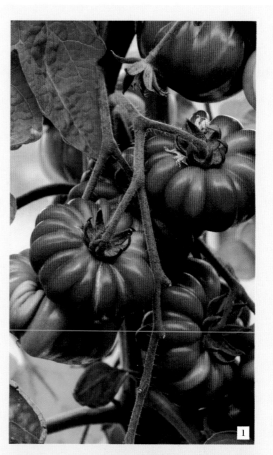

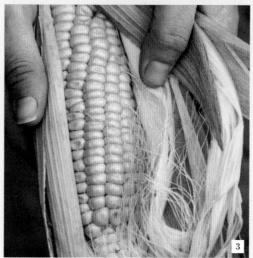

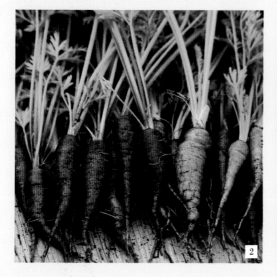

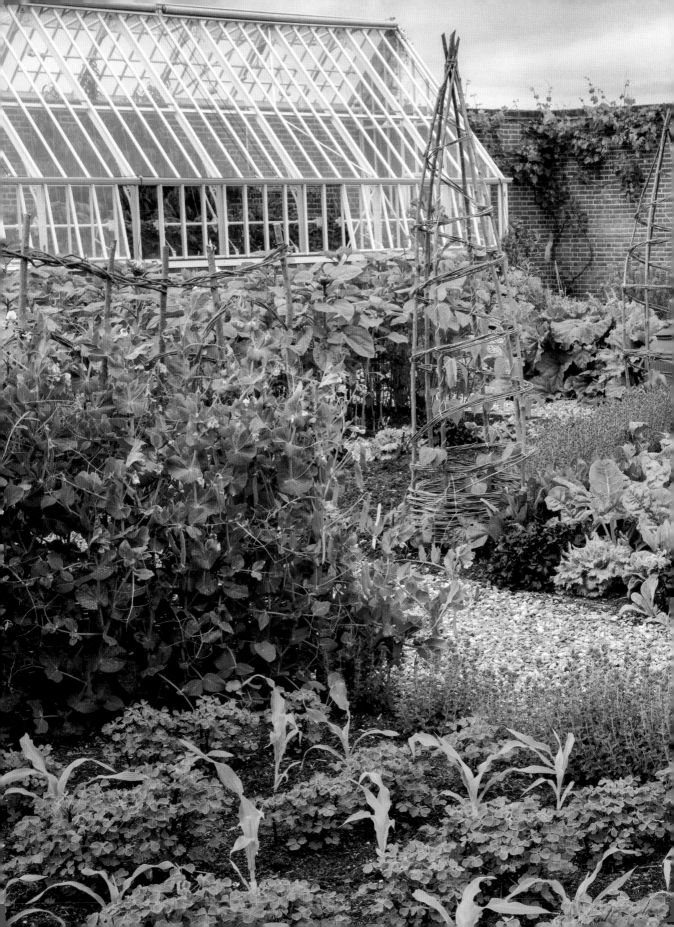

CHAPTER TWO

Vegetables & Fruit in Focus

*"Grow a variety of vegetables and fruit from different
botanical families to help increase diversity in your diet."*

"Members of the onion family help to protect us from cardiovascular disease, cancer and age-related problems, such as memory loss."

The onion family

Versatile, flavoursome and a key ingredient in many delicious recipes, onions, leeks and garlic pack a punch when it comes to our health, too, helping to lower blood pressure and reducing the risk of diabetes, heart disease and cancer.

I can't imagine life without onions and all their relatives (*Allium* species) – nearly every recipe I use starts with chopping onions and crushing garlic. We grow a wide variety of onions, leeks, garlic, shallots, spring onions (scallions) and chives for their flavour and health benefits. Generally thought of as basic culinary ingredients in most cuisines, they are exceptional from a nutritional perspective. While they are widely recognized as being a good source of vitamin C, it is actually their phytochemical content that makes them most interesting.

The pungent smell that is released when you cut into any type of allium is caused by sulphur compounds. These odorous phytochemicals are produced by the plant to deter animals and insects from eating them – it's a marvel our predecessors were able to overcome their natural reaction to this deterrent and discover how delicious these plants actually are. The sulphur compounds in onions have received lots of attention for their many health benefits, which include protection against cardiovascular disease, cancer and age-related problems, such as memory loss.

Alliums are also an important source of vitamin C, potassium, iron, selenium and polyphenols. The dietary fibre (fructans) they contain is an excellent fuel for our gut microbes too (see pages 16–19).

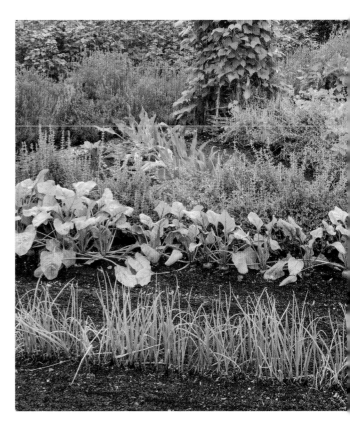

Add sulphur to the soil as a fertilizer when planting your onion crops: it increases the concentration of sulphur compounds in the bulbs, which are very beneficial to our health.

Onions
(Allium cepa)

GROWING FOR GUT HEALTH

- **Before you plant** Recent research shows that the phytochemical levels in onions are increased by adding mycorrhiza to the soil during planting. Mycorrhiza are fungi that live in the soil and promote good root growth. Sprinkle a small amount in the planting hole before planting or, if you practice 'no-dig' gardening (see page 27) and disturb the soil as little as possible, mycorrhizal and bacterial networks will develop naturally in the root zone.

- **Grow from sets** Grow your onions from sets rather than seed, as they result in 50 per cent more fructans, according to a German study. This is thought to be because onion sets have more advanced leaf development at the start of the growing season, and can take better advantage of available sunlight for photosynthesis.

- **Choose the best variety** If you have only space to grow one type of onion, opt for a red one. Red onions contain about three times more quercetin than white varieties, and have the added bonus of containing anthocyanins (see Health Benefits, opposite). Pungent varieties also have the greatest sulphur content.

- **Planting levels** Plant your onion sets out in mid-spring about 5–10cm/2–4in apart, with the tips of the sets just visible above the soil surface.

- **Feeding regime** Quercetin in onions increases in reaction to stressful growing environments, which is why they are better for you if grown in nutrient-poor soils. Nitrogen, in particular, should be avoided as it promotes leafy growth and reduces the amount of quercetin produced by the plants. However, applying sulphur as a fertilizer is very beneficial, and can double the sulphur compounds in the bulbs. Use sulphur powder, such as flowers of sulphur, when you plant out your sets.

- **Hope for a hot summer** Higher temperatures and drought also cause onions stress and induce them to increase their defensive chemicals. As a result, onions have higher levels of quercetin and anthocyanins during hot, dry summers. You can create similar benefits by minimizing the amount of water you give to your onion crop.

- **Protect outer scales** Retain valuable quercetin by protecting the outer layers when harvesting the bulbs, and remove as little as possible during cooking. More quercetin accumulates in older cells found in these outer scales because it protects against pest attack and damage from sunlight.

- **When to harvest** Studies have found that onions harvested later in the season have higher quercetin levels than those lifted earlier. This may be because the bulbs are exposed to more sunlight over the longer growing season.

- **Dry bulbs in the sun** Enhance the phytochemicals in your onions further by curing them in the sun. Harvest in a sunny week and lay the bulbs on the soil surface. Leaving them for a few days to dry in the sun maximizes their levels of quercetin and anthocyanins and also lengthens their storage life.

- **Storage and cooking tips** Storing onions in a cool, dark place doesn't have much impact on their nutritional value. In fact, some studies show phytochemicals actually increase during storage. Quercetin levels are also increased by sautéing or roasting onions, but do not cook them for too long, or boil them, as quercetin will leach into the water.

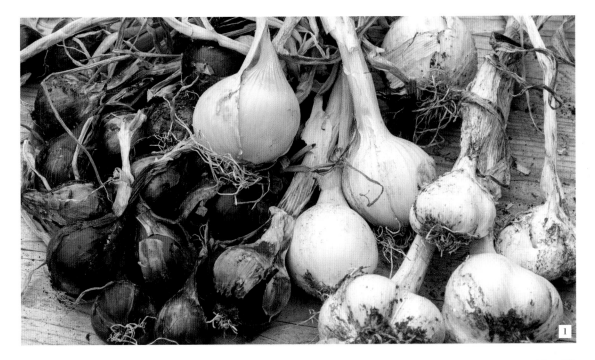

Health benefits

Onions are distinguished from other members of the allium family by their high levels of phytochemicals, namely quercetin, and in red varieties, anthocyanin is also present. Quercetin helps to reduce inflammation, relieves allergy symptoms, lowers blood pressure and reduces the risk of diabetes, heart disease and cancer. The quercetin levels in onions are actually higher than in most vegetables – they have three times more than broccoli. Onions are also good sources of the phytochemical saponin, which helps to lower cholesterol levels. In addition, they are an excellent source of the type of prebiotic fructans called fructooligosaccharides (FOS), which helps to maintain good gut health by fuelling our beneficial microbes (see page 19).

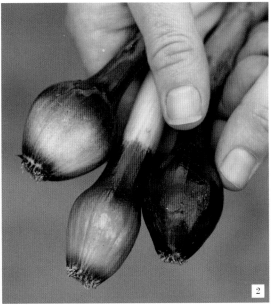

1. *Choose a range of onions, but grow red ones for the highest phytochemical content.* 2. *Grow spring onions from seed for a nutritious late-spring to early-summer crop.*

Leeks
(*Allium porrum*)

GROWING FOR GUT HEALTH

• **Sow seed** From early to mid-spring, sow seeds individually in pots or trays indoors – or multi-sow them in modules in groups of four or five seeds. You can also sow leeks directly outside from mid-spring onwards, once the soil has warmed up. Plant out the seedlings sown indoors from late spring to early summer, or thin those sown directly, and space them approximately 15cm/6in apart.

• **Water wisely** Scientific studies show that watering your leeks less frequently will increase the levels of prebiotic fibre, vitamins and minerals in the crops. However, too little watering may reduce your yield and cause the leeks to bolt early, so you need to strike a balance. A sensible approach may be to limit the plant's water intake by giving it in the mornings, rather than in the evenings when evaporation rates are generally lower and the ground will stay wet for longer.

• **Avoid pesticides** Recent studies show levels of sulphur compounds in leeks increase in response to pest attack (for example, from the leek moth). While you obviously want to avoid extensive pest damage, use organic methods and avoid pesticides to allow the plants to increase their own chemical defences naturally.

• **Increase sulphur** Apply sulphur fertilizer, such as flowers of sulphur, to increase the alliin content of your leeks (see page 47).

• **Balance your harvest** The period you harvest leeks also has an impact on their levels of polyphenols (see pages 20–21). If you harvest between midwinter and early spring, polyphenol and antioxidant levels are at their peak, while summer-harvested cultivars have the highest levels of fructans. This is because the plant stores energy in the form of fructans during periods of drought. To get the best of both worlds, sow some for summer harvesting and others to grow over winter.

• **Eat all parts** Different parts of the leek provide different benefits for your microbes. The white shaft is high in fructans, while the green leaves contain more polyphenols, due to their greater exposure to sunlight. So, for the maximum nutritional benefits, don't discard the green leaves when cooking.

• **Store and steam** The levels of polyphenols and fructans in leeks stay fairly constant in storage. The cooking method, however, does have a significant impact. Boiling leeks dramatically reduces the level of polyphenols as they are leached into the water, whereas steaming them has very little impact.

Health benefits

Leeks are underrated, both for their taste and the health benefits they offer. Planting them in summer fills me with confidence because I know I will be able to make a nutritious meal come the winter months. Dense with nutrition, leeks contain valuable prebiotic fibre, vitamins, minerals, polyphenols and sulphur compounds. They are an excellent source of the polyphenol kaempferol, which is notable for its anti-inflammatory and anti-cancer properties. Like garlic, leeks contain alliin, a sulphur compound that lowers blood cholesterol and helps protect against certain forms of cancer.

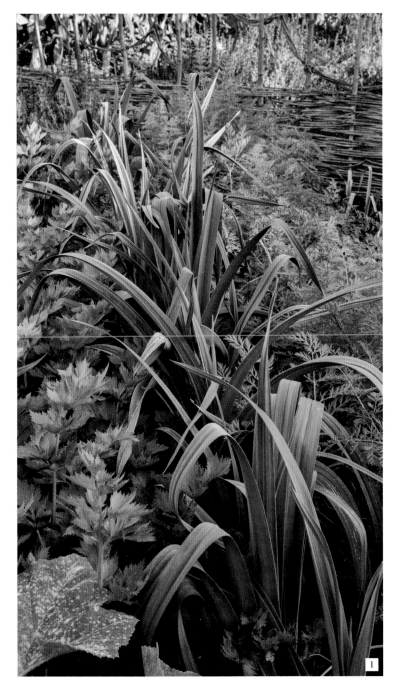

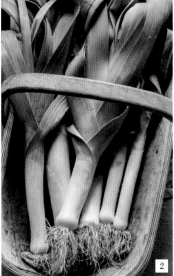

1. *Water your leeks less frequently to increase the levels of dietary fibre in the crops.* **2.** *Eat both the green leaves and the white shaft of the leek for optimal nutritional benefits.*

Garlic
(Allium sativum)

GROWING FOR GUT HEALTH

- **Choosing colour and variety** Select types of garlic that optimize nutritional values. Purple cultivars are higher in vitamin C, but white garlic is richer in phytochemicals (see pages 20–21). If you have space, why not grow both?

- **Growing garlic** Plant cloves directly outside from autumn until early spring. Plant approximately 15cm/6in apart and 5cm/2in deep and harvest from early to midsummer.

- **Food for thought** Sulphur increases the levels of sulphur compounds in garlic. It can be applied as a fertilizer in powder form, such as flowers of sulphur, during planting to enhance the nutritional value of your crops.

- **Be patient** Interestingly, the beneficial compound alliin (see Health Benefits, opposite) has been found to transfer from the leaves of garlic, where it accumulates during the early stage of growth, to the bulbs as they develop through the growing season. This means that leaving your garlic to mature fully before harvesting will maximize the alliin content in the bulbs, making them more nutritious.

- **Storing the goodness** Alliin levels increase during storage, so do not eat your garlic immediately if you want to maximize its nutritional value. Studies show the optimal antioxidant capacity of garlic is reached after 6–8 weeks in storage at about 20°C/68°F.

- **Take care when harvesting** Alliin is a very volatile substance, and is quickly released when physical damage is inflicted on garlic bulbs. To preserve this beneficial compound in the cloves try to avoid damaging them when harvesting and in storage.

Go wild for garlic

For an interesting addition to the vegetable garden, why not grow some of the naturally occurring wild species of garlic, since studies show the flowers and leaves of some of them have much higher levels of polyphenols than standard cultivated varieties. Rosy garlic (*Allium roseum*), hairy garlic (*Allium subhirsutum*), and Neapolitan garlic (*Allium neapolitanum*) can all be grown from bulbs planted in autumn. Mimic their native growing conditions by not enriching the soil, which will encourage them to accumulate more phytochemicals. They make a beautiful and tasty addition to salads or sprinkle them on stews and casseroles.

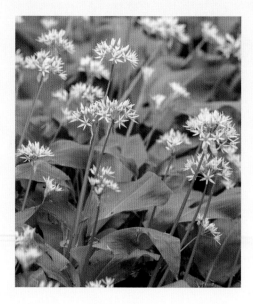

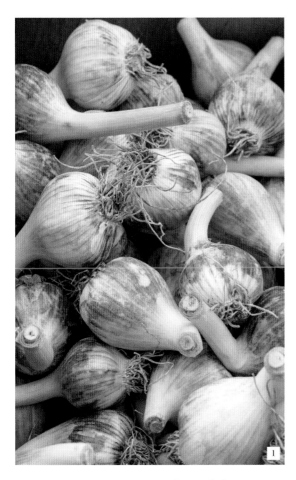

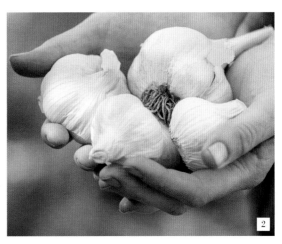

1. *Levels of sulphur compounds in garlic actually increase during storage.* 2. *Apply sulphur fertilizer to your garlic crops to enhance the pungency and phytochemical levels in the bulbs.*

Health benefits

The pungency of garlic is a reminder of its exceptional nutritional qualities. An excellent source of the B vitamins, vitamin C, and minerals, such as selenium, garlic is also a great source of prebiotic fructans, providing fuel for our gut microbes. However, it is the presence of alliin, the sulphur compound in garlic that produces its wonderful odour, which makes it so special nutritionally. When garlic is crushed alliin is converted by an enzyme into allicin. Allicin is not only a powerful antioxidant, protecting against heart disease and cancer, it is also a potent antibacterial, reducing harmful bacteria in the gut. In addition, allicin may help to lower blood pressure, reduce cholesterol levels and alleviate diabetes.

The carrot family

Modern science has shown that carrots cannot actually help us to see in the dark, but crops in this family are rich sources of phytochemicals that are responsible for good eye health, as well as helping to prevent cardiovascular diseases and cancer.

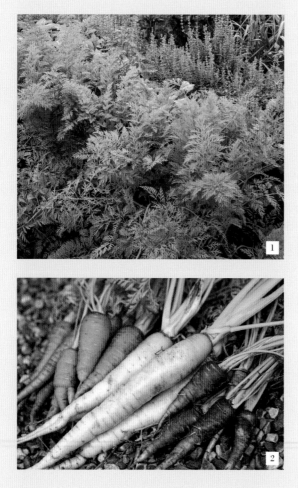

The carrot family is characterized by elegant flat-topped flowers (umbels). Many of these plants have underground taproots that store energy, including several edible crops, such as carrots, parsnips, celeriac and celery. The carrot family is also home to an array of culinary herbs, including chervil, coriander, dill, fennel, lovage, cumin, caraway and parsley. Rich in phytochemicals, including flavonoids and carotenoids, such as lutein, these herbs and crops help to promote good eye health, especially as we get older when our sight can degenerate.

Health benefits

Carrots have been cultivated for over 5,000 years and were first used as medicinal plants. They contain several important phytochemicals, including beta-carotene, which the body converts to vitamin A, lutein, and lycopene (in red carrots). Lutein is important for eye health, while lycopene, an antioxidant also found in tomatoes, protects against heart disease and cancer, and promotes healthy skin – it may even help to prevent sunburn. Purple carrots are also rich in anthocyanins. In addition, carrots contain various B vitamins, vitamin K and potassium, and are good sources of fibre.

1. *Carrots grown in full sun have higher levels of carotenoids.*
2. *Purple carrots have more polyphenols than orange or white ones.*

Carrots
(Daucus carota subsp. *sativus)*

GROWING FOR GUT HEALTH

- **Choose a colour** Surprisingly, carrots haven't always been orange – until the seventeenth century they were purple, yellow or white. Dutch carrot breeders then selected an orange form to please their monarch, William of Orange, which is now the most ubiquitous type. However, not all political decisions are for the best. Studies have found that purple carrots have the highest overall antioxidant activity and the best balance of phytochemicals, such as carotenoids and polyphenols, and they also contain anthocyanins (see pages 20–21). It's important not to limit yourself to purple carrots, though. Yellow carrots are great sources of lutein and red carrots contain high levels of lycopene (see Health benefits, left).

- **Sow outside** Sow carrots directly outside between mid-spring and midsummer. When the leaves appear, thin to approximately 5cm/2in apart and cover the crop with fine mesh to prevent carrot root fly from attacking it.

- **Hot it up** Research has found carrots grown in hotter temperatures have higher levels of carotenoids – growing them over summer will increase these phytochemicals.

- **Harvest when young** The phytochemical content of carrots is higher in younger roots and declines quickly in the first three months of growth, so harvest your carrots as baby veg.

- **Forget fertilizers** Plant fertilizers, such as boron and calcium, used to boost yields of commercially grown carrots, have a negative effect on polyphenols. The reason is probably because they strengthen plants' cell walls, while untreated carrots

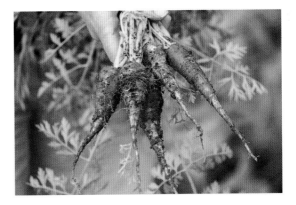

Young carrots have the highest levels of phytochemicals, while adding olive oil to carrot dishes helps us to absorb their nutrients.

that are more susceptible to injury have a greater need for phytochemical protection. The best advice is not to mollycoddle your crops with extra minerals.

- **Goods in store** The phytochemical content of carrots generally increases in storage: carotenoid levels remain stable for months in cold storage.

- **Skin deep** It's best not to peel carrots before cooking because the polyphenols are most concentrated in the skin and decrease gradually towards the core. This is because the outermost layer of the root is the most vulnerable to damage.

- **Cook for health** The availability of carotenoids increases when carrots are cooked because the raw roots have tough, fibrous cell walls that are difficult to digest. We can only convert about a quarter of the beta-carotene in them into vitamin A. Cooking breaks down the cell walls, releasing these compounds for us to absorb. Steaming is one of the best cooking methods, as the phytochemicals can leach into the water when carrots are boiled.

"Beetroot is packed with nutrients and has special health benefits, such as increasing blood flow and muscle efficiency and reducing tiredness."

The beet family

Beetroot and its relatives, chard and spinach, are among the most nutritious vegetables you can grow. Rich in vitamins, minerals and phytochemicals to boost your health, there are a number of simple growing methods you can try to increase the benefits even further.

I've recently been growing more and more plants from the beet family because they tend to be what growers call 'good doers' – easy to cultivate, relatively free of pests and diseases, and high yielding. A fairly diverse family, its members include chard, beetroot, amaranth, spinach, and some more unusual crops, such as agretti, orach, Mexican tree spinach and Aztec broccoli.

The beet family crops are packed with polyphenols, vitamins and minerals, which offer a range of health benefits. Beetroot contains nitrate, which helps to improve blood flow and reduces tiredness, while its close cousin Swiss chard offers similar benefits. Most people know that spinach is nutritious, but you may not know that it contains 40 per cent more health-boosting polyphenols than cabbage, and 70 per cent more than lettuce.

Here, I've focused on the more commonly cultivated vegetables from the group, but I would encourage you to try growing other family members as well, if you haven't already, as they are really delicious and packed with nutrients. Agretti has a wonderful crunchy texture, very similar to samphire, while the leaves of Mexican tree spinach have an incredible pink bloom that indicates their high levels of polyphenols. You're also very unlikely to find these more unusual varieties to buy in the supermarket, but seeds are available from specialist suppliers, so by growing your own you can include greater diversity in your diet without spending a fortune.

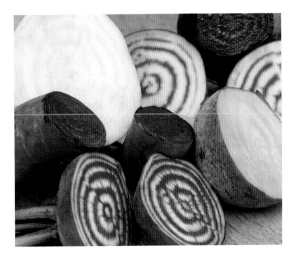

Beetroot contains an unusual type of polyphenol called betalain, which has powerful antioxidant properties.

Beetroot
(Beta vulgaris)

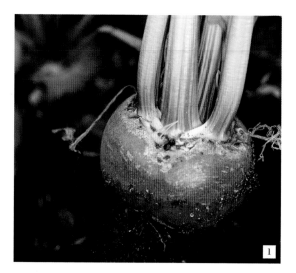

GROWING FOR GUT HEALTH

- **Best for betalain** The polyphenol betalain, present in beetroot, comes in two forms: betacyanins, which give the roots the deep red colour they are famous for, and betaxanthins, found in yellow or orange beetroots (see Health benefits, opposite). White beetroot tastes sweet but does not contain any beneficial betalain, while stripy cultivars have none in the white parts of the roots. Try growing a range of different colours for diversity's sake, but if space is limited, opt for a variety with a strong red colour. My favourite for flavour is 'Cylindra', which has unusually long taproots, rather like a carrot.

- **No-fuss sowing** Sow seed outside in the ground at 10cm/4in intervals from mid-spring to late summer, then thin to the strongest seedling when the leaves emerge. Alternatively, sow seed in groups in modules under cover in spring – thin groups to four or five seedlings and plant out together when the weather warms up, from late spring.

- **Grow outside** The betalain content of beetroots grown outside is 25 per cent higher than those grown under cover. This could be due to increased stress when plants are exposed to the elements, such as higher levels of sunlight, drought, or greater differences between day and night temperatures. Most people grow beetroot outside anyway, but this may be useful for anyone tempted to do otherwise.

- **Keep cool and dry** Levels of polyphenols, such as betalain, in beetroot are at their highest in cooler weather – temperatures over 25°C/77°F reduce its production. Grow beetroot during the cooler times of the year, ideally sowing in early spring or late in the growing season when it's not as hot to reap the benefits. Research also shows betalain and nitrate is increased when plants are water stressed, so keep plants on the dry side.

- **Eat the skins** The concentration of polyphenols, such as betalain, is much higher in the skin than in the flesh of the roots, so eat the skin if possible.

- **Eat the leaves** The leaf stalks (petioles) of beetroot, especially red stalks, contain a third type of betalain called isobetalain. The leaves are a great source of phytochemicals too, so add some to your dishes to access these benefits. I also save beetroot seedling thinnings to use in salads and sandwiches.

- **Store well** Beetroot's phytochemical levels remain relatively constant when stored in cool conditions.

- **Raw goodness** The phytochemical content is highest in raw beetroots. Grate or slice them in salads or, if cooking, sauté or steam the roots rather than boiling, which results in the phytochemicals leaching into the water. I also roast my beets whole with the skins on to retain the goodness.

Health benefits

Beetroot is a highly versatile vegetable, usually eaten for its sweet roots, although it also has nutritious edible leaves. The roots are a rich source of vitamins A and C, and the leaves contain minerals such as calcium and iron. However, it is beetroot's high inorganic nitrate content that has received the most media attention in recent years. Studies have found that this type of nitrate helps to improve blood flow and muscle efficiency, and reduces fatigue – research showed that when athletes ate beetroots as wholefoods, as opposed to taking the nitrate in a supplement form, they improved their performance in endurance trials.

Beetroot has also been prized since Roman times as an aphrodisiac, due to its boron content, which is said to increase sex drive. It offers a variety of phytochemicals too. The roots' intense colour comes from betalain, which is a type of polyphenol and potent antioxidant with anti-inflammatory properties. In a study of 23 vegetables, beetroot was found to have the highest overall betalain content. Scientists are keen to explore other health benefits this polyphenol may offer, such as how it affects cognitive functioning as we age, and its impact on insulin resistance, cancer and liver damage.

1. Growing beetroot early and late in the season increases its polyphenol levels, which rise in crops grown in cooler temperatures. 2. Eat both the leaves and the roots of beetroot for the greatest diversity of phytochemicals.

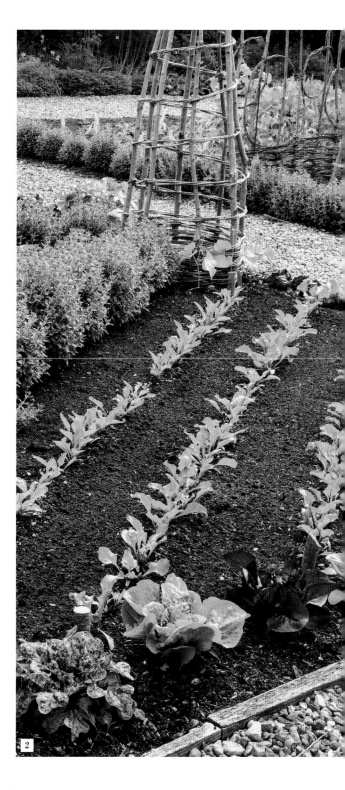

Swish chard
(*Beta vulgaris* subsp. *cicla* var. *flavescens*)

GROWING FOR GUT HEALTH

• **Select colourful stems** Less research has been conducted into the cultivation of Swiss chard than beetroot, but there is one very useful study that compares the betalain content of different coloured stems. Betalain is the beneficial polyphenol that is also in beetroot (see page 52). The highest content was found in chard with purple stems, followed by red, yellow and, lastly, yellow/orange. So purple

varieties are the best overall for betalain and are an excellent choice for home-growers. There are some fantastically lurid cultivars, such as 'Magenta Sunrise', which has almost luminous purple stems. However, yellow varieties should also not be ignored, as they contain the highest levels of betaxanthin (see page 52). Seed suppliers usually sell 'Rainbow Chard' mixes, which are a great cost-effective option for growing a diversity of different-coloured chard in a small garden.

• **Sow successively** Sow seed outside or indoors in modules from mid-spring to midsummer. I sow two to three seeds at 35cm/15in intervals and thin to the strongest seedling. Despite their Mediterranean origins, the plants are very hardy and will stand outside all through the winter.

• **Year-round harvesting** Swiss chard is a year-round crop that can be harvested throughout the summer and winter months. Cut the leaves close to the base of the stem. Frequent harvesting will also encourage fresh new growth to develop. Although it is highly nutritious all year, the phytochemical content is likely to be at its highest under conditions of stress during the cooler periods of the year and if watering is kept to a minimum. Ideally grow chard on free-draining, sandy soil to reduce moisture retention.

• **Cook with care** Steam lightly or microwave chard to prevent the phytochemicals leaching out into the cooking water. Eat the stems too, as they contain the important phytochemical betalain and are also a rich source of dietary fibre. The green leaves are delicious raw in salads or can be lightly cooked like spinach. They contain other types of phytochemicals, as well as vitamins and minerals, and are highly nutritious (see Health benefits, left).

Health benefits

Swiss chard is a great source of vitamin K – just 100g/3½oz provides over three times the recommended daily dose – as well as being rich in vitamins A and C, minerals and fibre. Closely related to beetroot, it has a similar phytochemical profile, and contains the polyphenols betalain, betacyanin and betaxanthin (see page 52), which determine the different colour pigments found in the leaf stem. There's a whole range of brightly coloured varieties to choose from, including purple, red, orange, and yellow. White chard is also popular, but, like white beetroot, it is an albino form that lacks betalain. I must admit the white-stemmed variety 'Fordhook Giant' is a favourite of mine, but there are much more nutritious varieties you can grow.

The green leaves of Swiss chard also contain different types of beneficial phytochemicals with important antioxidant properties that help to protect against cancer, cardiovascular diseases and inflammation.

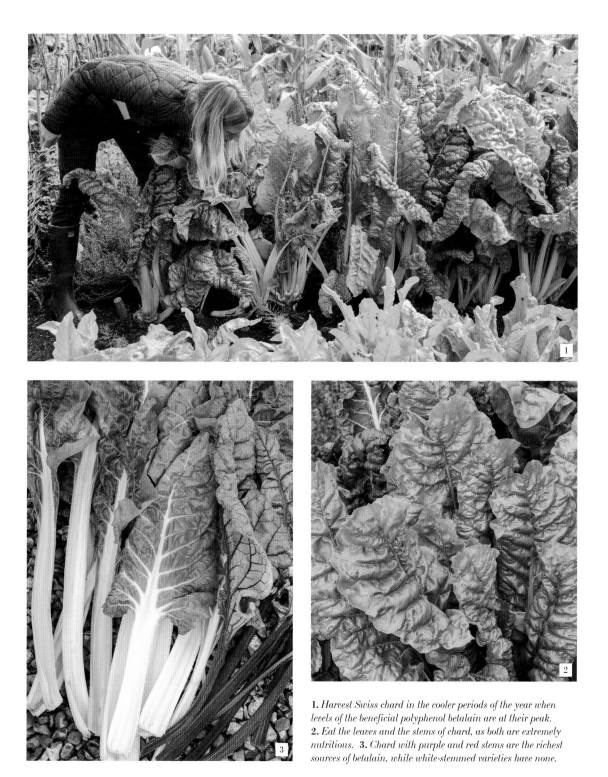

1. Harvest Swiss chard in the cooler periods of the year when levels of the beneficial polyphenol betalain are at their peak. 2. Eat the leaves and the stems of chard, as both are extremely nutritious. 3. Chard with purple and red stems are the richest sources of betalain, while white-stemmed varieties have none.

Spinach
(Spinacia oleracea)

GROWING FOR GUT HEALTH

- **Tough defences** Select varieties of spinach bred for disease resistance, which will naturally have higher phytochemical levels as a defence mechanism. These are usually described in seed catalogues as having downy mildew resistance; examples include 'Palco' and 'Amazon'. Red-veined or red-stemmed varieties, such as 'Reddy', are also worth growing, as the pigmentation indicates the presence of anthocyanins, another valuable phytochemical (see pages 20–21). Also try growing the climbing Malabar spinach (*Basella alba*), which is a different genus of plant to regular spinach but produces a prolific crop of nutritious leaves, and will add diversity to your diet.

- **Try two sowings** Sow seed outside in mid-spring for early summer harvesting, and then again in midsummer for a winter or early spring harvest. Sow three to four seeds at intervals of 10–15cm/ 4–6in and do not thin the seedlings – just pick off the leaves as needed and the plant will then produce more a few weeks later.

- **Pick leaves when almost mature** The levels of phytochemicals in spinach vary, depending on when you pick it. Harvest the leaves when they are bigger than baby leaves but before they expand into fully mature leaves, as the phytochemicals are over 30 per cent higher at this stage of growth.

- **Keep plants stressed** Give spinach a long growing season to maximize the phytochemicals. Studies show that if you sow spinach in autumn, it's best to wait until the following spring to harvest it, when the level of phytochemicals and antioxidant activity are much higher. Spinach sown in early autumn and harvested in mid-winter had only half the phytochemical content of crops picked the following spring. This suggests spinach grown over a longer period is subjected to more stress factors, which increase its nutrient value.

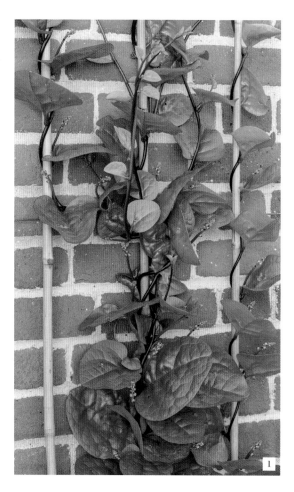

1. The easy-to-grow climber, Malabar spinach, will help to increase the diversity in your veg plot. *2. Pick spinach leaves when semi-mature for the highest polyphenol levels.*

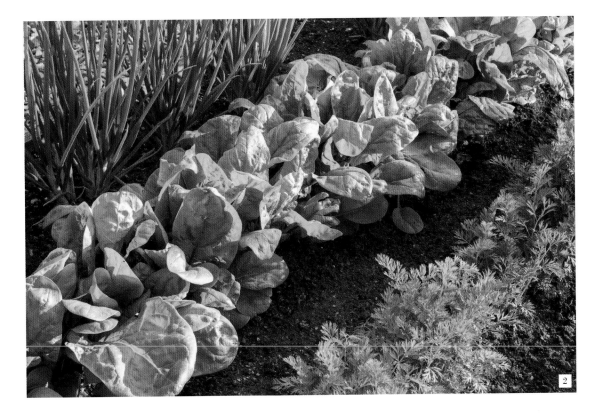

2

• **Use natural fertilizers** Scientists have discovered phytochemical levels in spinach can be increased by adding plant-based fertilizers, such as seaweed extract and protein extracts from legumes. These biostimulants increase phytochemicals that help the plant to defend itself against pests and diseases, while simultaneously increasing its nutritional value. Like many gardeners, I've been using seaweed extract for years, so it's gratifying to discover it has such tangible health benefits.

• **Eat fresh** Spinach is best eaten fresh because the phytochemicals quickly decline when it is stored in the dark conditions of a refrigerator. Ideally, eat yours picked straight from the garden.

• **Cook lightly** Cooking spinach can dramatically reduce its phytochemical levels. Boiling reduces them by over 40 per cent as the nutrients leach into the water, so either lightly steam the leaves or cook them in the microwave to minimize losses.

Health benefits

In the US in the 1930s, there was a 33 per cent increase in spinach sales, largely thanks to the spinach-devouring popular cartoon character Popeye. Although the theory that eating spinach will turn us all into Popeye may be a myth, this leafy vegetable is one of the most nutritious we can grow. Very high in dietary fibre, minerals (especially calcium, manganese, and iron), and vitamins A, B, C, and E, spinach is also a rich source of the carotenoid, lutein. Lutein reduces the risk of cataracts and protects against declining eyesight as we age. Spinach has 40 per cent more phytochemicals than cabbage and 70 per cent more than lettuce, so it is well worth including more of it in your diet if you can.

The asparagus family

Nothing heralds the new growing season like the tender, green stems of asparagus which, contrary to popular belief, are very easy to grow. Plant in full sun to optimize its health benefits and this nutrient-rich crop will reward you year after year.

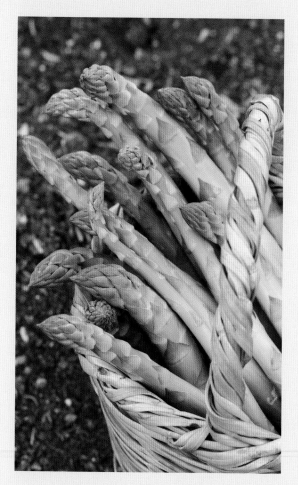

Nutritious asparagus is a rich source of fibre, sulphur compounds, vitamins and phytochemicals.

> "Packed with fibre and phytochemicals, asparagus is one of the best crops to grow for your gut health."

The asparagus season often marks the start of the really prolific growing period in the vegetable grower's calendar. It's definitely one of my favourite times of the year, often coinciding with the tulips and apple blossom in full bloom in the walled garden.

For some reason asparagus has a reputation for being difficult to grow, but that is unwarranted. Provided the initial groundwork is done and the site cleared of pernicious weeds, asparagus is very little bother. It requires some patience, however, as the spears will only be ready to harvest after the third year of growth, but the plants will then supply you with delicious stems year after year, with minimal input required from you.

Asparagus
(Asparagus officinalis)

GROWING FOR GUT HEALTH

- **Go for green or purple** Breaking with the tradition of purple and red vegetables containing the most polyphenols, green asparagus has actually marginally more phytochemicals overall. However, purple asparagus spears do have a significantly higher rutin content, which is known to improve blood circulation, but it is quite a close-run thing nutritionally, and either of these two varieties would make a good addition to the vegetable garden, so make room for both if you can.

- **Prepare the ground** Choose a sunny or partially shaded site for your asparagus plants and remove any perennial weeds before planting. Plant crowns of asparagus about 45cm/18in apart in mid-spring, and cover them with roughly 7–8cm/3–3½in of soil or organic matter, such as home-made compost. Mulch the beds from late autumn to early spring every year with home-made compost or well-rotted manure. Asparagus needs a few years to establish, and the spears should be ready to pick in the third year after planting.

- **Let plants see the light** White asparagus is not a specific variety, but you can produce it by covering the crop to block any sunlight. This prevents the asparagus from photosynthesizing (making energy from the sun's rays) and producing chlorophyll, which gives the spears their green colour. Asparagus is managed in this way to reduce bitterness and, while it has a wonderful mild flavour, this is at the expense of most of its nutritional value. White asparagus has much lower antioxidant activity than green or purple forms, with no rutin and nearly half the polyphenols. So, if you want to optimize your phytochemical intake, take the covers off and expose your crops to the sun.

- **Harvest the whole shoot** Perhaps unsurprisingly, the highest levels of dietary fibre are found in the bases of the stems, so try cutting lower down the shoots for more fibrous fuel for your microbes. Rutin, on the other hand, is found in the highest concentrations at the tips of asparagus spears.

- **Eat fresh and cook lightly** Asparagus does not store well. To optimize its nutritional value, eat it as quickly as possible after harvesting and cook the stems lightly by steaming. Boiling is especially damaging, as up to 50 per cent of the polyphenols are leached into the cooking water.

Health benefits

Asparagus is very nutritious and an excellent source of vitamins, especially vitamin K and folate. Fans of asparagus will also be pleased to know that it's one of the best vegetables to grow for gut health, as it is a good source of prebiotic fibre, which promotes a healthy digestive system (see pages 16–19). It's also an excellent source of phytochemicals that help to protect against cancer, heart disease, inflammation and allergies, as well as having a positive effect on the immune system and decreasing cholesterol levels. Purple asparagus contains anthocyanins, too, which have powerful antioxidant qualities (see pages 20–21). Asparagus also contains sulphur compounds that can make your urine smell (although apparently not everyone can detect it), but have many health benefits, including promoting healthy skin and hair.

"Members of the sunflower family are valued for their high fibre content, which provides a great source of fuel for our gut microbes."

The sunflower family

Encompassing thousands of plant species, the sunflower family is home to a wide range of delicious, nutritious vegetables, including lettuces, chicory and globe artichokes, which provide fibre to feed our gut microbiota, as well as a host of vitamins and phytochemicals.

The sunflower family is one of the largest and most diverse botanical families with over 20,000 naturally occurring species. As well as the large yellow blooms we associate with sunflowers, this group includes edible plants, such as lettuces, which need no introduction, chicory, and globe artichokes. Many of these crops are excellent sources of fructans, the fermentable fibre that provides fuel for our gut microbes (see pages 16–19).

Chicory has been a popular vegetable since 4,000BC, when the ancient Egyptians used the root to produce chicory coffee. Research today shows it also has many benefits for our gut health. Globe artichokes are among the most architectural and striking plants in the edible garden. They produce beautiful purple blooms, but if you harvest the flowerheads just before they open, they will reward you with more antioxidants than wild blueberries.

Jerusalem artichokes are very closely related to sunflowers and at first glance the plants look similar, with their bright yellow blooms. Unlike their close relative, however, these artichokes have underground tubers that are rich in fibre and nutrients.

Other edible varieties in this diverse family are dandelion greens, yacon and cardoons, which are also worth growing to increase the diversity in your diet. It may seem mad to cultivate dandelions, which we know as a weed, but the leaves offer a welcome nutritious treat before other plants emerge in spring.

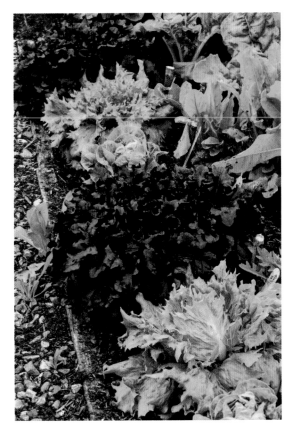

The sunflower family is one of the most diverse in the botanical world. The most popular edible member is the humble lettuce, but there are many more unusual varieties to grow, such as yacon and cardoons, that will increase the diversity in your diet.

Globe artichokes
(Cynara cardunculus)

GROWING FOR GUT HEALTH

• **Opt for purple hues** There are many different varieties of artichoke to choose from – some have green heads, others are tinged with purple – and there is considerable variation between different cultivars and their polyphenol content. One study into six common commercial varieties found the popular 'Violet de Provence' had the highest overall phytochemical content, while levels of the fibre, inulin, were particularly high in 'Romanesco'.

• **Sow seed or buy plants** Sow seed in pots or modules indoors in mid-spring, or buy young plants and plant them outside in spring or autumn. Artichokes require little maintenance but ensure these large perennial plants are set out at 80–90cm/32–36in intervals to give them space to grow. They will produce flowerheads year on year.

• **Add beneficial fungi** Mycorrhiza are fungi that reside in the soil and have a symbiotic relationship with plants. Recent research shows that by adding mycorrhiza to the soil during planting, the phytochemicals were increased in globe artichokes by over 50 per cent. Alternatively, by practising 'no-dig' gardening (see page 27), and disturbing the soil as little as possible, mycorrhizal and bacterial networks will naturally develop in the root zone.

• **Go for the heart** The total polyphenol content in globe artichokes increases by up to six times from the outer bracts towards the inner bracts (leaf-like sections that protect the flower) and the artichoke heart (the receptacle of the flower). The heart is, of course, the best part of the artichoke. Now you can savour it even more in the knowledge that you are also providing your gut microbes with a gourmet treat and improving your overall health. Don't

Health benefits

The key phytochemicals in globe artichokes are the flavonoids apigenin and luteolin. Both of these compounds have been found to help reduce the risk of cancer and apigenin may also protect against Alzheimer's disease. They are not found in many foods, which makes artichokes well worth growing. Artichokes also contain a special form of inulin which is super-effective as a prebiotic (see pages 16–19), fuelling the bacteria *Bifidobacteria* and *Lactobacillus*, which are very beneficial to gut health.

discard the outer bracts, though, as some specific types of polyphenols, including apigenin, do the opposite and increase towards the outer edges.

• **Cold and light** Combining cold temperatures and high light levels is optimal for polyphenol production in globe artichokes. Exposing the plants to strong sunlight is particularly effective, increasing the levels of polyphenols in the hearts of the flowerheads, so ensure your artichokes are in a sunny spot and don't worry if they're subjected to the cold.

• **Keep in store** The phytochemical content of artichoke heads actually increases by up to 50 per cent when they are stored for a week or two. Generally, however, the quality of artichokes quickly deteriorates after it is harvested, rapidly losing its firmness. It may be worth leaving your artichokes in the refrigerator for a few days after harvesting to accumulate phytochemicals, but don't leave them for too long or they will lose their succulence.

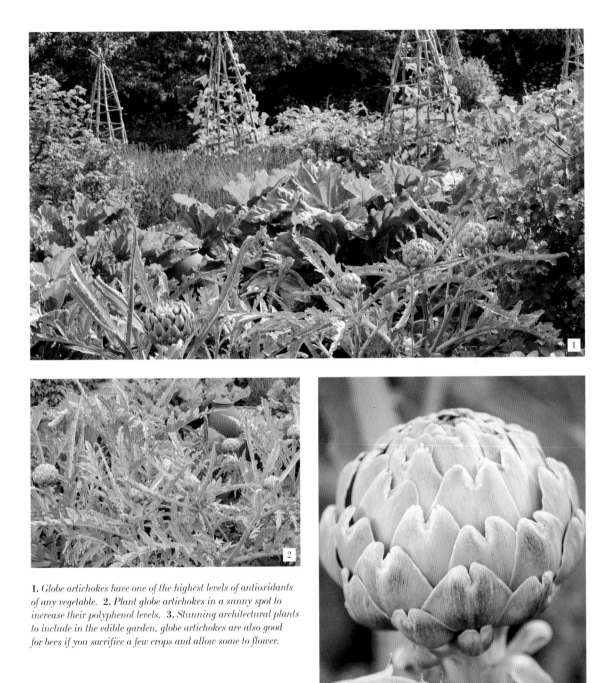

1. *Globe artichokes have one of the highest levels of antioxidants of any vegetable.* 2. *Plant globe artichokes in a sunny spot to increase their polyphenol levels.* 3. *Stunning architectural plants to include in the edible garden, globe artichokes are also good for bees if you sacrifice a few crops and allow some to flower.*

Jerusalem artichokes
(Helianthus tuberosus)

GROWING FOR GUT HEALTH

- **Choose late varieties** Different cultivars of Jerusalem artichoke have varying levels of the fructans, inulin (see page 19). A Danish study tested a range of cultivars and found those with late-maturing red tubers had the highest inulin levels. So, although any Jerusalem artichokes will be excellent sources of this prebiotic fibre, choose late red and purple cultivars for their microbe-boosting benefits.

- **Plant out in spring** Plant tubers out in mid-spring about 30cm/12in apart and 10–15cm/4–6in deep. Plants grow very tall, so cut back to 1.5m/5ft in midsummer to avoid wind damage. Removing the flowerheads will also help with tuber development. Jerusalem artichokes grow in a wide range of

conditions, but prefer a sunny site and free-draining soil. These perennial plants produce tubers year after year, but be warned, they can be very invasive. If left in the ground and not harvested the tubers will quickly colonize an area; each one has the potential to produce 75–200 more tubers each year. This is wonderful for harvesting, but keep them in check. Ideally plant them in a raised bed or dedicated area of the garden where they cannot escape.

- **Autumn harvest** Crops will start to mature from autumn onwards as the foliage dies back. Inulin levels peak around early to mid-autumn as the tubers mature (depending on the variety); levels then gradually decrease until the following spring, so harvest in autumn for the best health benefits. Closer to spring, the plant converts inulin into fructose (natural sugar), which the plant is able to use for energy in the new season of growth.

- **Warm summers maximize benefits** Temperature has been found to have a significant effect on the inulin content in Jerusalem artichokes: the warmer the growing conditions, the more inulin is produced. This is perhaps because there is a link between tuber development and environmental stress caused by drought or temperature shifts.

- **Eat without delay** Inulin levels decrease over time when tubers are stored. In tests, Jerusalem artichokes kept for over four months showed a marked decline in inulin levels – another good reason to grow your own and make sure you reap the freshest, most inulin-rich vegetables available.

- **Baking is best** The highest levels of inulin are found in raw Jerusalem artichoke tubers. If you prefer them cooked, bake them in the oven rather than boiling them to retain the most beneficial fibre.

Health benefits

Inulin, the prebiotic fibre in Jerusalem artichokes, stimulates the growth of beneficial bacteria in the gut, and protects against inflammatory disorders and diseases, such as cancer and diabetes. The roots are also rich in B vitamins and thiamine, which is critical to the functioning of the nervous system and muscles. They are delicious but have the nickname of 'fartychokes', so be careful how many you eat in one meal.

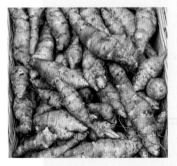

Dandelions
(*Taraxacum*)

GROWING FOR GUT HEALTH

- **Sow indoors or out** Sow seed under cover or directly outside in the ground in mid-spring, as soon as the soil warms up sufficiently. Plants need little care or attention after sowing and they can be harvested as a cut-and-come-again vegetable by simply snipping off the leaves you need and waiting for a new crop to appear a week or two later.

- **Treat them mean** While there have not been many studies of dandelions, it is sensible to assume that by applying some environmental stress, such as growing them in poor soil, exposing plants to full sun, and minimizing irrigation, the polyphenol content of these plants will be increased.

- **All dandelions are not equal** One word of caution: seed catalogues sometimes sell seed for 'Italian dandelions'. These are not, in fact, true dandelions but a very close relative, *Cichorium intybus* (common chicory). They are equally nutritious, and contain high levels of prebiotic fibre and phytochemicals, so do grow them as well, but be aware they're a different species of plant. I grow a red-ribbed form of this plant, which has the added polyphenol, anthocyanin (see pages 20–21).

···

AMAZING DANDELION FACT

As an interesting aside, dandelions are unusual in that they can produce seed without the need for pollination. One of a select number of plants able to do this, the seeds they develop are clones of the mother plant. This is partly why dandelions are able to spread across your garden so quickly.

···

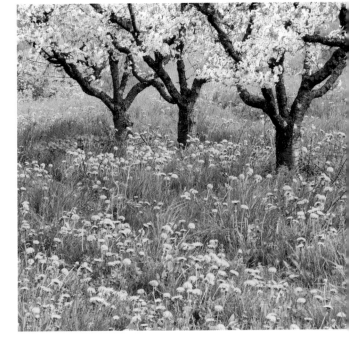

Cultivated dandelions make a nutritious crop, rich in fibre, which promotes good gut health, and a range of phytochemicals.

Health benefits

All parts of the dandelion plant are edible and the prebiotic fibre, inulin, is found in both the leaves (12–15 per cent) and roots (25–40 per cent). Dandelions also contain an array of different phytochemicals, including lutein, which supports good eye health, and apigenin, quercetin and luteolin, which are all potent antioxidants with anti-cancer and anti-inflammatory properties.

Chicory
(*Cichorium intybus*)

GROWING FOR GUT HEALTH

- **Red is best** When choosing which chicory cultivars to grow for the highest levels of polyphenols, colour is a clear indicator. Red raddichio cultivars, including 'Rossa di Verona', 'di Chioggia' and 'Rossa di Treviso', have over six times as many polyphenols as green varieties, while popular variegated cultivars, such as 'Variegata di Castelfranco', rank somewhere in between the two. Also grow root chicory, *Cichorium intybus* var. *sativum,* for its high inulin content (see page 19).

- **Summer sowings** Sow chicory from early to midsummer indoors and plant out, spacing the seedlings approximately 30cm/12in apart, from mid- to late summer. Chicory is a great vegetable for successional planting after earlier crops have been harvested. It can be used as a cut-and-come-again vegetable too: cut stems back to their bases and they should resprout for two or three harvests. It is also possible to force chicory, which means excluding light from the plants to produce yellow, sweeter leaves. However, covering the crop reduces the plants' phytochemical content, which is stimulated by sunlight.

- **Going to seed** Chicory is biennial, which means it flowers and sets seed in the second year. A study showed the seed has the highest phytochemical content and antioxidant activity. Leave a few plants to set seed to use in salads or as a garnish. Chicory flowers look attractive in the garden too.

- **Grow in ridges** The same study also found sowing root chicory in ridges in the soil produces higher yields of inulin. Although this method is normally associated with ploughing on a farm, it's easy to recreate in a garden. Simply mound the soil into inverted V-shaped ridges and sow or plant on the tops of them. The ridges will create a better aerated soil structure for root development.

- **Harvest times** When chicory roots are left in the ground, they convert inulin into another form of fructans (oligofructose), which is a more readily available form of energy for the plant to use. Both types of fructans help to fuel our gut bacteria, so harvest them over time to maximize the benefits.

- **Store away** Storage doesn't seem to have much of an impact on the levels of polyphenols of chicory, but antioxidant activity decreases over time.

- **Heat the leaves** Levels of polyphenols increase when the leaves are cooked, except when boiled, which has a detrimental effect. Microwaving is best, resulting in up to 25 per cent more phytochemicals. Also retain and eat the outer leaves, as studies show these are richer in polyphenols because they have been subjected to more environmental stress.

Health benefits

Chicory leaf is an excellent source of polyphenols that help to protect against cancer and inflammation. Red varieties also contain anthocyanins, powerful antioxidants, and are especially useful in winter when other sources, such as berries, are out of season. Root chicory, *Cichorium intybus* var. *sativum*, has similarly high inulin levels to Jerusalem artichokes (see page 64); it is 98 per cent inulin when dried and is commonly used in prebiotic supplements.

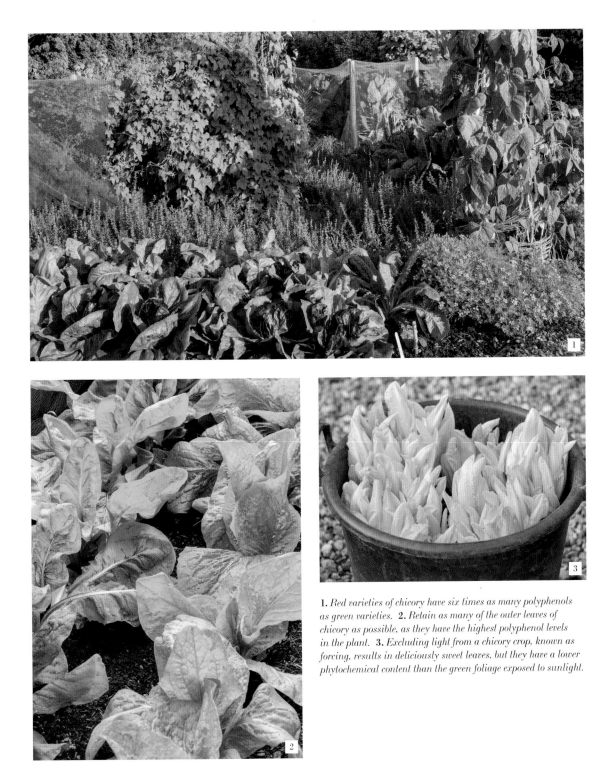

1. *Red varieties of chicory have six times as many polyphenols as green varieties.* 2. *Retain as many of the outer leaves of chicory as possible, as they have the highest polyphenol levels in the plant.* 3. *Excluding light from a chicory crop, known as forcing, results in deliciously sweet leaves, but they have a lower phytochemical content than the green foliage exposed to sunlight.*

Lettuces
(Lactuca sativa)

GROWING FOR GUT HEALTH

- **Top of the charts** There is a huge disparity in the level of phytochemicals found in different varieties of lettuce. A study into five of the most popular types of lettuce and their respective polyphenol content showed that 'Lollo Rosso' had the most, followed by red oak leaf, green oak leaf, romaine and, lastly, iceberg. In fact, the red 'Lollo Rosso' had an astonishing 31 times more than the iceberg. This is because phytochemicals accumulate in the leaves that are exposed to the elements, including sunlight, cold temperatures and pest and disease attacks. Therefore, open-headed varieties are likely to have higher levels of polyphenols than those with tightly held, protected leaves, such as iceberg. When choosing varieties to grow, bear these principles in mind and opt for open-headed lettuces, especially red ones.

- **Sow in succession** Sowing some lettuces every few weeks from spring onwards allows me to comfortably grow three crops a year. Sow seed under cover from early spring onwards, or directly outside in the ground from mid-spring to midsummer. Ideally, grow in full sun or part-shade in free-draining soil and space plants approximately 25cm/10in apart. Lettuces are remarkably hardy and will withstand quite low temperatures into winter.

- **Keep plants cool** Lettuces that are grown at low temperatures have significantly higher levels overall of polyphenols and anthocyanins. Studies show that when grown in day and night temperatures of 13°C/55°F and 10 °C/50°F, crops had over 15 times more anthocyanins than lettuce grown at 30°C/86°F and 25°F/77°F. Similarly, the total polyphenol content was 11 times more in the lettuce grown in cool conditions. For gardeners, this suggests that lettuce grown during cooler periods of the year, in spring and autumn, is likely to be much more nutritious.

- **Grow outside** A study analyzing the polyphenol content of lettuces grown in glasshouses and outside showed all crops grown outside had higher polyphenol levels, with 43 times more flavonols than the glasshouse-grown plants. Again, environmental stresses stimulate the plants to increase their protective phytochemicals. Given that most of the lettuces bought at the supermarket are grown in polytunnels, cultivating your own outside has a major nutritional benefit.

- **Eat the outer leaves** More quercetin is found on the outer leaves of lettuces; quantities decrease gradually towards the centres of the heads, so retain as many older leaves as possible. In fact, if you harvest the leaves of your lettuces gradually, picking the outer leaves rather than harvesting whole heads, you can reap these greater nutritional benefits over the course of the season. The carotenoids in lettuces are also more easily digested if good-quality oil is added to them during preparation.

- **Store for health** The phytochemicals in lettuces increases during storage, but, despite these health benefits, the crop also deteriorates quickly after harvesting in terms of taste and flavour. It is important to find a balance between offsetting the benefits in terms of nutrition against losses in the sensory quality of your lettuce leaves.

- **Diversity matters** Lettuces are not very nutrient dense so try to grow other leafy salad crops too, such as mustards, oriental greens, wild rocket or watercress, which have stronger flavours and much higher levels and diversity of phytochemicals.

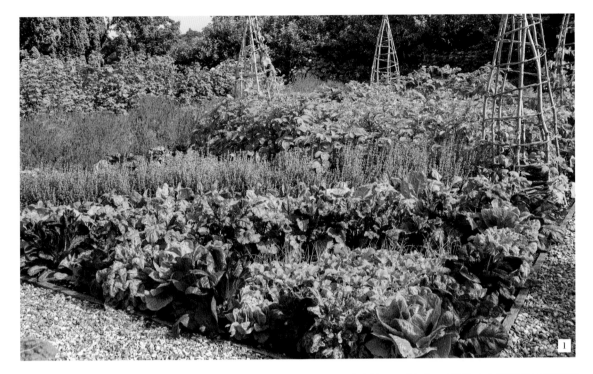

Health benefits

Lettuces have relatively low levels of dietary fibre, but they are good sources of vitamins, especially beta-carotene, which the body converts to vitamin A, as well as vitamins K and C. The leaves also contain folate, manganese and iron. Phytochemicals in lettuces depend on the variety, but they include lutein, rutin, quercetin and kaempferol, which protect against cancer, heart disease, inflammation and allergies. Some also contain epicatechin, which supports muscle growth, and red types are a source of anthocyanins (see pages 20–21).

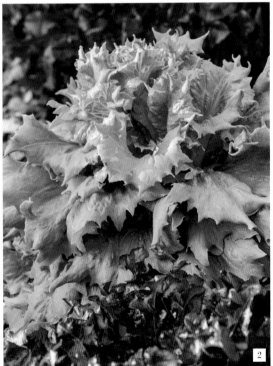

1. There are dozens of lettuce varieties to choose from, but loose-leaved, red varieties offer the best health benefits. 2. The outer leaves of lettuces have the highest quercetin levels, which help to protect against cancer, heart disease and allergies.

"Grow members of the cabbage family for tasty, nutritious treats during the lean periods in spring and autumn."

The cabbage family

A diverse group of crops, this family includes kale, Brussels sprouts, radishes and rocket, as well as cabbages. All are excellent sources of special sulphur compounds that promote good gut health and also protect us against cancer and cardiovascular disease.

The cabbage family is a robust group that includes hardy leafy greens, such as kale, cabbages and Brussels sprouts, together with hot and peppery radishes, horseradish and rocket. Oriental greens, such as pak choi, mizuna and komatsuma, and kohlrabi are also in this group. Known collectively as brassicas, many of these crops are cool-season plants and will quickly bolt in the heat.

Cabbages, Brussels sprouts, broccoli, cauliflower, kohlrabi, kale and collard greens are all variants of one species, *Brassica oleracea*, which in its wild form grows by the Mediterranean coast. The mature plants of these different cultivated brassicas look radically different from one another, but the seeds and seedlings are almost impossible to tell apart. This demonstrates the power of human ingenuity in that we have be able to breed one species over the centuries to create such delicious diversity.

So what makes brassicas good for us? All of these vegetables contain sulphur compounds called glucosinolates, which are responsible for the slightly bitter aftertaste some of these plants have. We are unable to absorb glucosinolates in their pure form, but when we chop, chew or otherwise physically injure brassicas, these compounds react with an enzyme in the plants to produce sulforaphane, which we can absorb. Sulforaphane increases the beneficial bacteria in the gut and helps to protect against various forms of cancer and heart disease, while supporting a healthy brain and digestive system.

Brassicas also contain polyphenols that help to prevent cancer, and red forms, such as red cabbage, are sources of anthocyanins, which have good antioxidant properties. Surprisingly, carotenoids, the yellow, red and orange pigments found in other crops, are also present in some brassicas. Beta-carotene is converted to vitamin A in the human body and promotes healthy eyes and skin.

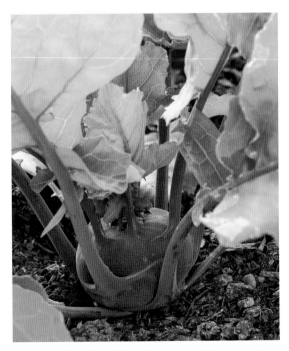

Grow kohlrabi early and late in the season and choose purple varieties for the highest levels of phytochemicals.

Broccoli
(Brassica oleracea Italica Group)

GROWING FOR GUT HEALTH

- **Wild wonders** Wild relatives of brassica crops have been found to contain more glucosinolates than their cultivated cousins – a study showed levels are increased two or three times by crossing a standard cultivar with a wild type. This so-called 'super broccoli' is marketed under the name of Broccoli 'Beneforté', but unfortunately it is not possible to buy and grow the seeds of this variety at this time because, controversially, it has been patented by the chemical giant Monsanto. This could set a worrying precedent, restricting access to valuable health-related genetic resources.

- **Choose a cool spot** Sow seed from mid-spring to early summer, outside or under cover. Space plants approximately 45cm/18in apart in a prepared bed in sun or part-shade – in hot and dry weather plants have a tendency to bolt. Protect plants from cabbage-white butterfly by covering with netting or using an organically certified biological control, such as *Bacillus thuringiensis.*

- **Water wisely** Limit the amount of water you give to your broccoli plants and ideally grow them on free-draining soil to increase their levels of glucosinolates and polyphenols – researchers in Italy found polyphenols were increased by 35 per cent when broccoli plants were exposed to drought. However, in a dry season, seriously limiting irrigation will have a negative impact on yield and may cause the broccoli to bolt early, so you will need to do some watering, but try not to overdo it. In hot, dry weather, give your plants a good soak every few days, rather than a daily sprinkling.

- **Select the right fertilizer** Standard gardening advice often advocates feeding broccoli with nitrogen. I used to follow this faithfully, applying chicken manure to the soil before planting to boost nitrogen levels. However, by not applying nitrogen fertilizer, you can increase polyphenols by up to 80 per cent. Adding sulphur, on the other hand, increases glucosinolate levels and polyphenols – apply flowers of sulphur to your soil when planting. Seaweed feed is another excellent option. Field studies show that it creates at least a two-fold increase in the levels of polyphenols and glucosinolates in the broccoli florets.

- **Nutritious sprouts** Levels of glucosinolates in broccoli vary depending on the plant's stage of maturity. For example, three-day-old broccoli sprouted seeds have 10–100 times the amount of glucosinolates as mature florets. So, if space is limited, why not grow small amounts of broccoli

Health benefits

As I write this section, I'm in the process of weaning my six-month-old baby. I'm keen to make sure she eats green vegetables and broccoli is already a favourite. It's such a joy to cut the broccoli fresh, steam the florets and feed them to my baby, knowing how nutritious they are. As well as offering a rich source of glucosinolates (see page 71), some types could potentially offer even greater benefits. All types of broccoli are excellent sources of vitamins A, C and folate, carotenoids, calcium, iron and dietary fibre. Purple sprouting broccoli also contains health-boosting anthocyanin and higher antioxidant levels than green varieties.

1. Fertilize broccoli plants with sulphur to increase the levels of glucosinolates, which help to prevent cancer and heart disease and benefits the brain and digestive systems. 2. Eat your freshly harvested broccoli as quickly as possible after harvesting.

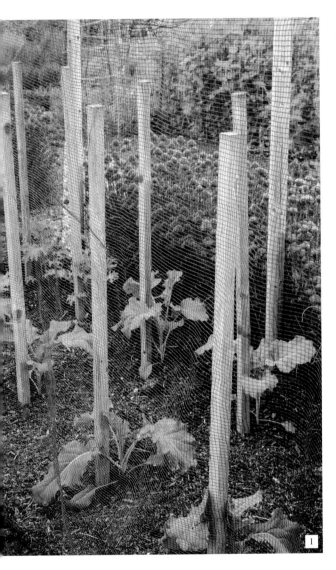

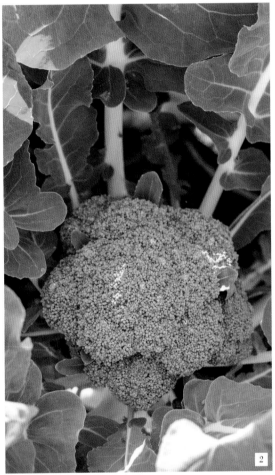

sprouts to gain the same nutritional benefits as the mature plant? (See the Sprouting seeds project on pages 152–53 for further advice).

• **Fresh is best** The nutrients in broccoli rapidly deteriorate after harvesting and typical commercial transport and storage conditions could reduce levels of glucosinolates by up to 80 per cent. Growing your own crop and eating it soon after harvesting is definitely the best way to optimize the nutritional value of broccoli.

• **Eat the stems** While the broccoli florets are tender, the stem is higher in dietary fibre. Include both next time you cook it, rather than discarding the base. I find freshly harvested broccoli tastes completely different to supermarket vegetables in any case, and you can slice through the stems like butter. The best way to preserve the glucosinolates in broccoli is to eat it raw, or steam or microwave it. Boiling has a particularly detrimental effect, not just on the glucosinolates but also the vitamin C content and protein in the florets.

Brussels sprouts
(Brassica oleracea Gemmifera Group)*

GROWING FOR GUT HEALTH

- **Bitterness is best** The level of glucosinolates in Brussels sprouts varies widely according to the cultivar (see Health benefits, opposite). Most people prefer sprouts with a mild flavour, but it is actually the bitterness of the glucosinolates that makes them so nutritious. Recent plant breeding programmes have focused on selecting varieties with lower levels of this sulphur compound, and consequently they have a lower nutritional value, but as gardeners we can opt for varieties known to be more beneficial to our health. Recent scientific studies have found that common cultivars, such as 'Dominator' and 'Doric' have especially high values of glucosinolates, while red varieties, including the cultivar 'Rubine', have the added bonus of containing anthocyanins.

- **Sow indoors** You can sow Brussels sprouts seed outside in a sunny bed from mid- to late spring, but I prefer to sow mine indoors, where I can more easily protect my plants from pests until they are established. Plant outside once the seedlings have at least three to four true leaves. Leave a space of 60cm/24in between the plants and add a stake next to each one – Brussels sprouts are tall plants, have a long growing season and will need support, especially in the winter. It may be necessary to also protect your plants from cabbage-white butterfly by covering the crop with netting or using an organically certified biological control, such as *Bacillus thuringiensis*.

- **Sunny side up** Plant your Brussels sprouts in full sun to increase their phytochemical levels. Recent research has shown that brassica plants produce higher levels of these beneficial compounds when subjected to stress from UV radiation.

- **Boost the plant microbiota** Micro-organisms in the soil help Brussels sprouts to absorb sulphur compounds. Like humans, plants host a community of micro-organisms, called the plant microbiota (see pages 26–27). Associated microbes around the roots help the plant to absorb nutrients, including sulphur compounds. So, by helping our Brussels sprout plants to develop healthy and extensive root systems we can also increase their uptake of sulphur from the soil, which in turn increases the plant's production of glucosinolates. Minimize soil disturbance by not digging it, and mulch with plenty of organic matter, such as home-made compost. This will create a beneficial environment for the plant roots and the plant microbiota to thrive.

- **Add sulphur** Like other brassicas, Brussels sprouts benefit from an application of organically certified sulphur fertilizer, such as flowers of sulphur, during the growing season. This leads to an increase in glucosinolates in the crops.

- **Harvest in spring** Research has shown that the highest levels of glucosinolates are found in Brussels sprouts in the spring. The longer day length, higher levels of sunlight and warmer temperatures at that time of the year result in greater phytochemical levels than if you harvest in mid-winter, when daylight hours are shorter and temperatures lower. It doesn't mean you have to miss out on the Christmas sprouts, just make sure you save a few for later in the year as well.

- **Fry or steam** Boiling reduces the polyphenols and antioxidant activity in Brussels sprouts, so next Christmas why not try stir-frying or lightly steaming them instead, which research shows preserves their health-boosting compounds. They are also delicious roasted with garlic, olive oil and salt.

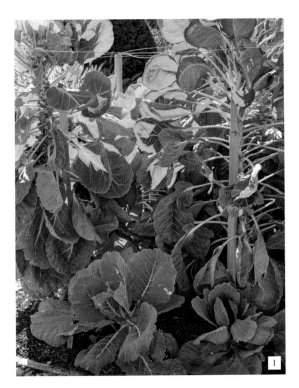

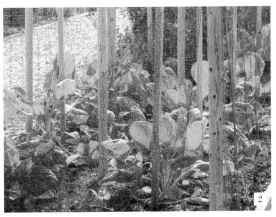

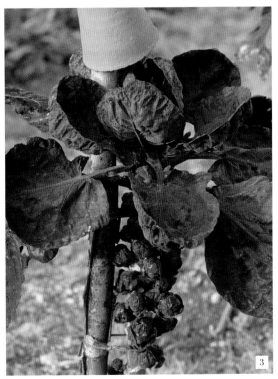

Health benefits

In 2014 a man raising money for charity pushed a Brussels sprout up the highest mountain in Wales using just his nose. It took four days and 22 sprouts (presumably because they kept rolling off). Now I have your attention, let me tell you about their nutritional value. In a study of 42 different brassica cultivars, Brussels sprouts were found to contain the highest level of glucosinolates, with their incredible cancer-prevention qualities. They are also notable for their carotenoids and polyphenol content (see pages 20–21). In a study of several varieties of broccoli, cabbages, cauliflower, Chinese cabbage and Brussels sprouts, they had the second highest overall polyphenol content, and twice that of cabbages, cauliflower and Chinese cabbage.

1. Brussels sprouts have more cancer-preventing glucosinolates than any other common brassica vegetable. *2. Grow your Brussels sprouts in full sun to increase polyphenol levels.* *3. Red Brussels sprouts are available to grow from seed and are rich in anthocyanins, with their potent antioxidant properties.*

Kale
(Brassica oleracea Acephala Group)

GROWING FOR GUT HEALTH

- **Back to black** A study of 62 cultivars of broccoli, cabbage and kale found varieties of black kale, also known as Cavolo Nero kale were extremely rich in glucosinolates – one cultivar of Cavolo Nero had 26 per cent more than were found in broccoli. Don't ignore the other types of kale, though. Red kale is a great source of anthocyanins, especially in the winter when berries and other fruit are not in season (see pages 20–21).

- **Sow twice a year** There are two possible sowing periods for kale. Sow directly outside in a sunny spot, or indoors, in mid-spring for summer harvesting, and again in midsummer for a winter crop. Spring-sown kale will continue to stand throughout the winter but the plants can become straggly. Space plants 50cm/20in apart and protect them from cabbage-white butterfly by covering with netting or using an organically certified biological control such as *Bacillus thuringiensis.*

- **Pick when mature** A couple of studies have found carotenoid levels are much higher when the leaves are fully open and mature. Antioxidant activity in mature leaves is 22 per cent higher than in young baby leaves. However, do not harvest leaves that are wilting or browning, as the carotenoid levels drop quickly as the foliage starts to deteriorate.

- **Grow inside or out?** Levels of sunlight and temperature both affect carotenoid and glucosinolate production in kale plants. Studies show kale harvested in summer has the highest concentration of carotenoids where crops are grown under protection, such as a plastic sheet. This is thought to be because too much sunlight exposure can damage carotenoid compounds.

In winter, the reverse is true: kale grown outside has a higher carotenoid content than crops grown under protection because the covered crops have restricted exposure to the limited sunlight available.

- **From plot to plate** Carotenoids quickly degrade in high temperatures. After cutting the leaves, transfer them to a refrigerator straight away. Do not leave them out to wilt in the sun and eat them as quickly as possible, ideally on the day you harvest them.

- **Raw truths** For the highest nutritional value, eat your kale raw or steam it lightly to maximize polyphenols levels – boiling will leach them into the water. A study of red and green curly kales showed red kale lost 28 per cent of the polyphenols during cooking, and green kale lost 48 per cent.

Health benefits

In recent years kale has been widely lauded as a superfood. In the US, there is even a 'National Kale Day' in October to celebrate its health benefits. Rich in dietary fibre, calcium, vitamins C and K, and iron, it has high antioxidant levels and is a good source of glucosinolates and polyphenols. Kale is particularly notable for its carotenoids, such as lutein and zeaxanthin, which protect against age-related eye disease. Beta-carotene levels in kale are significant too – in a study of 63 cultivars of broccoli, cabbages, kale and cauliflower, kale ranked the highest overall. Kale is also a source of flavonoids, and red varieties contain anthocyanins (see pages 20–21).

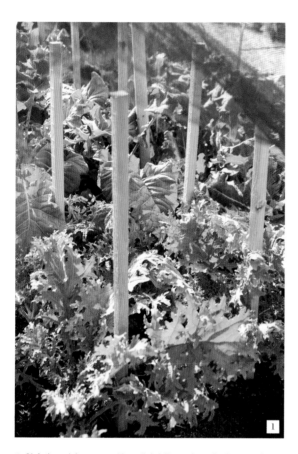

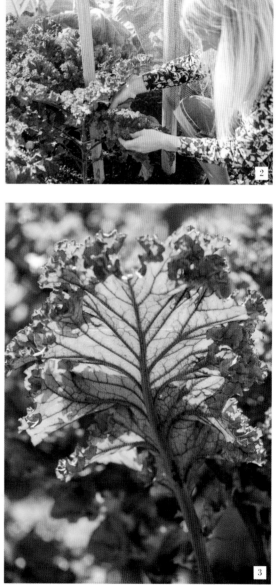

1. *Kale is a rich source of beneficial fibre, glucosinolates and carotenoids.* 2. *Harvest when the leaves of kale are mature for optimum nutrition.* 3. *Red kale has additional anthocyanins which become more prevalent during cool weather. The colour of many cultivars turns a deeper red as winter progresses.*

Cabbages
(Brassica oleracea Capitata Group)

GROWING FOR GUT HEALTH

• **Three colour options** A study looking at the polyphenol content and antioxidant capacity of red, white, and Savoy cabbages found red cabbages had the highest total levels, largely due to their anthocyanin content. Red cabbages have over five times more polyphenols than white, and over three times more than Savoy cabbages. However, Savoys have the highest beta-carotene content, and white cabbages contain the most lutein, which promotes good eye health, so grow all three types if you can.

• **Sow for two harvests** Sow seed indoors or directly in the ground in late spring for autumn or winter harvests, and again from mid- to late summer indoors or outside for a spring harvest. I find it best to sow plants indoors, where I can protect the seedlings from pest attack, planting them out once they have become more established. Space plants 40–50cm/16–20in apart, and protect them from cabbage-white butterfly by covering with netting or using an organically certified biological control, such as *Bacillus thuringiensis*.

• **Reduce watering** As with other members of the brassica family, reducing irrigation tends to increase glucosinolates in cabbages; levels are particularly high when crops are not watered while the heads are forming.

• **Food from the sea** Seaweed fertilizer has recently been shown to increase the phytochemical content in plants. A trial into cabbages fed with seaweed extract showed total polyphenol levels were increased by up to two times, and flavonoids by a similar degree (see pages 20–21). Seaweed extract can be applied to crops either as a foliar feed or as a soil drench.

• **Optimum harvest times** Young cabbages have a higher phytochemical content than mature plants so don't leave them sitting in the ground for too long before harvesting them. In addition, cabbages planted in spring or early summer (for an autumn to winter harvest) have a 40 per cent higher content of polyphenols, glucosinolates and antioxidant activity than autumn-planted varieties. This makes sense because those harvested later in the year have been exposed to a long summer of high temperatures, drought and UV levels, which cause phytochemicals to accumulate.

The time of day for harvesting also makes a difference. Levels of glucosinolates will actually vary over a 24-hour period, reaching a maximum in the afternoon. This was shown in study of kale and cabbages, but presumably also applies to other members of the brassica family too.

• **Outer leaves are best** Cabbages' outer leaves contain twice the glucosinolates of the inner leaves, so try to discard as few as possible when you're preparing one. Additionally, the tougher outer leaves contain more dietary fibre, so they are definitely worth adding to your dishes.

• **Light touch** Cook cabbages lightly by microwaving or steaming to preserve the phytochemical content.

• **Savour the sauerkraut** Sauerkraut is one of the most popular ferment recipes, with good reason, as the process of fermentation creates live cultures of good bacteria for your gut. Fermenting your home-grown vegetables also increases their polyphenol content. Studies show that making sauerkraut from home-grown cabbages increases its total content by 30 per cent – even more reason to ferment your crops (see page 180 for a recipe).

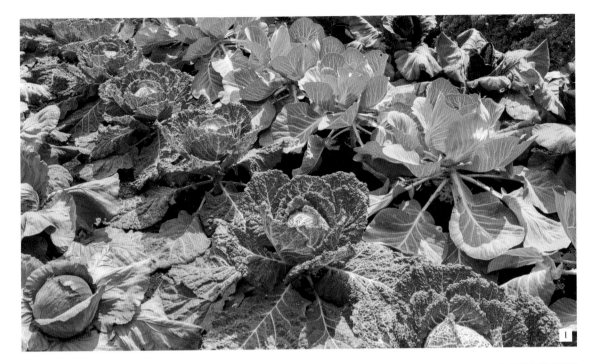

Health benefits

Although cabbages seem to be less popular than they once were, I've been growing more of them in recent years, partly because they are so useful in fermentation recipes, and because I've discovered how good they are for our health. Cabbages are a rich source of vitamins C and K, and iron. Up to 40 per cent of a cabbage is also made up of dietary fibre – ensuring healthy bowel movements and providing fuel for our gut microbes. Like other brassicas, cabbages contain glucosinolates (see page 71), with their anti-cancer effects, plus unusual compounds called phytosterols, which have a phenomenal effect on lowering cholesterol by blocking our absorption of it in the digestive tract. Red cabbages contain anthocyanins, too, which help to maintain a healthy heart.

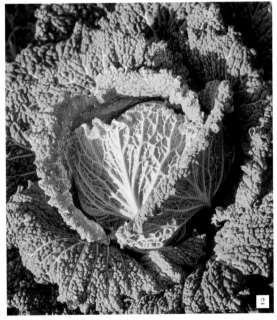

1. *Grow different varieties of cabbage, if you have space, to benefit from their different types of phytochemicals.* 2. *As ingredients for fermentation recipes, freshly harvested cabbages are far superior to those from the supermarket, due to their high moisture content.*

Cauliflower

(Brassica oleracea Botrytris Group)

GROWING FOR GUT HEALTH

- **Brightly coloured bonus** A study of 12 types of highly pigmented purple vegetables, including cauliflower, carrots, aubergines, potatoes, onions and cabbages, found that purple cauliflower ranked number one overall for total polyphenol content and antioxidant activity, due to the high anthocyanin content (see pages 20–21). However, glucosinolates are highest in green and 'Romanesco' cultivars, while the lowest levels are in purple and white cauliflowers, with the green types containing up to 11 times more than the traditional white. So take your pick or grow all of them if you have space.

Health benefits

Where I grew up in Cornwall cauliflower was always called 'broccoli' and broccoli was called 'calabrese'. I've no idea why, but for all you non-Cornish folk we'll stick to calling it cauliflower. Why should we be growing it? Cauliflower is high in dietary fibre and vitamins B and C, and it is a good source of carotenoids (see pages 20–21) and glucosinolates (see page 71). Cauliflowers come in different, sometimes shocking, colours, including yellow, green and purple, all of which are more nutritious than white forms.

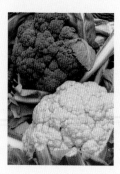

- **Plant closely** Sow seed indoors or outside in sunny beds from mid-spring to early summer. I sow plants indoors in small pots to better protect the seedlings from pest attack and plant them out once the seedlings are more established (when they have formed at least three or four true leaves). Space plants 30–35cm/12–14in apart, or at a density of about 8–9 plants per square metre/yard. This is closer than is normally recommended, as scientific studies have shown that greater planting density increases the crops' polyphenol levels. Protect your cauliflowers from cabbage-white butterfly by covering the crop with netting or using an organically certified biological control such as *Bacillus thuringiensis*.

- **Keep heads clear** Commercial growers often break a leaf to cover the heads of cauliflowers, which protects them from sunlight and keeps the florets white. Do not be tempted to do likewise, as this technique significantly reduces the amount of glucosinolates, anthocyanins, carotenoids and the antioxidant activity in the cauliflowers.

- **Feast on florets** The florets of cauliflower are 60 per cent higher in glucosinolates than the stalk, although the stem is a rich source of dietary fibre, so it's best to eat both.

- **Sprouting good health** Like broccoli, sprouting cauliflower seeds causes a massive increase in glucosinolate levels – a whopping 10–100 times more than is found in mature plants.

- **Do not boil** Boiling cauliflower causes the biggest loss of nutrients and phytochemicals, as they are leached into the water. Steam, microwave or stir-fry the florets instead for the best health benefits.

Radishes
(*Raphanus sativus*)

GROWING FOR GUT HEALTH

- **Pick a type** There are hundreds of radish varieties to choose from, including the Asian daikon or mooli radishes, black winter radishes, and even sweet radishes, such as the Chinese 'Watermelon' and green 'Shawo Fruit'. Adding a few more types of radish to your veg plot will increase the diversity in your diet for much of the year.

- **Easy does it** Sow seed directly in the ground in a sunny spot from mid-spring to late summer. The distance between plants depends on the type of radish. Traditional round radishes or French breakfast types can be thinned to about 5cm (2in) apart. Daikon or winter radishes are best sown in late summer and need much more space – thin to 20–30cm/8–12in apart. Radishes can be susceptible to flea beetle attack, so cover with an extra-fine mesh to protect them, if needed.

- **Sun and light** A study into 13 cultivars of radishes grown in three different altitude locations in Korea found glucosinolate levels were up to 33 times greater in the highest location. This is thought to be due to the environmental stress caused by the high UV levels and the differences between night and day temperatures. Other studies that show phenolic content increases with higher levels of sunlight exposure. For those of us not planning to move to a mountain location, simply grow radishes in full sun and aim for more exposed locations.

- **Sprouting success** Radish sprouts have nearly four times the levels of glucosinolates, and nearly seven times the amount of polyphenols, as mature radishes. Sprout seeds of radish 'Sango', which are an excellent source of anthocyanins.

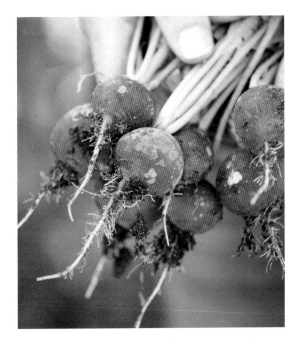

Radishes are a quick and easy, nutritious crop, very useful for planting between larger crops that take longer to mature.

Health benefits

Radishes' antioxidant activity helps to enhance health and prevent chronic diseases. There are many different types available to the home-grower, apart from the popular French breakfast and pink globe varieties, that offer a range of other benefits. All radishes contain glucosinolates and polyphenols, including anthocyanins (see pages 20–21) in the skins of red and purple types, while black radishes have the highest levels of sulforaphane (see page 71).

The squash family

Try growing a range of pumpkins, courgettes and other squashes to aid gut health and provide nutritious meals for many months of the year. They offer a rich source of phytochemicals that promote good eye health and protect against cancer and heart disease.

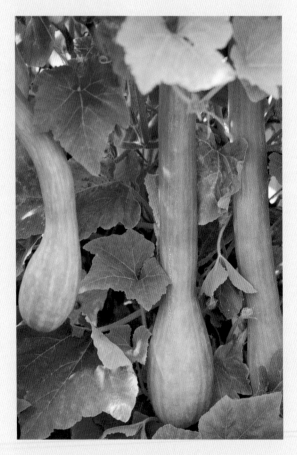

Grow the beautiful 'Tromboncino' squash up a support, such as trellis or horizontal wires fixed to a wall or fence, for prolific quantities of their elongated, nutrient-rich fruits.

The squash family contains both summer- and winter-fruiting varieties, offering a nutritious feast for most of the year. We grow a wide range of both, and love testing new varieties. Summer squashes include the popular, heavy-cropping courgette, and many other varieties. The first year I had an allotment I grew about ten courgette plants just for me; a classic newbie error, but I was still ecstatic with my crop.

Other types include yellow crookneck and patty pan squashes, which have a lovely nutty flavour. The unusual 'Tromboncino' is always a talking point, with its huge, elongated fruits, like swans' necks. It is best picked young, but I can never resist allowing a few to become marrows, just to see how large they will grow. Winter squashes include three distinct species: the classic culinary pumpkins and squashes (*Cucurbita maxima*), acorn squashes and traditional Halloween-style pumpkins (*Cucurbita pepo*) and butternut squashes (*Cucurbita moschata*). If space is limited, try growing trailing types up supports.

Nutritionally, squashes are an excellent source of carotenoids, including alpha- and beta-carotene, which the body converts to vitamin A. Summer squashes are also high in B vitamins, and all types are rich in dietary fibre, vitamins C and folate, manganese, and potassium. The type of squash you choose and the way you grow and harvest them impacts on their nutritional value. Winter varieties, in particular, store for a long time, providing a valuable source of nutrition when there are few other crops to eat.

Courgettes (zucchini)
(Cucurbita pepo)

GROWING FOR GUT HEALTH

- **Colour matters** Choose dark green varieties of courgettes for the highest carotenoid content (lutein and beta-carotene). Yellow courgettes rank second for their phytochemical content, but white varieties of summer squash (such as the patty pan types) have virtually no carotenoids and, therefore, are much less beneficial from a health perspective.

- **Give them space** Sow seeds indoors in late spring. I sow two seeds per 9cm/3½in pot and thin to the strongest seedling. Plant out when all risk of frost has passed. Give plants plenty of space to grow, leaving at least 1m/3ft between them. Courgettes are often affected by powdery mildew in hot, dry summers, but if this happens simply remove affected leaves to limit the spread of the disease.

- **Small bounty** Baby courgettes are better for you than larger fruits. A recent study showed small courgettes have 100 per cent more polyphenols and antioxidant activity than medium or large fruits.

- **Flower power** The flowers of courgettes are now a popular edible, but they perish rapidly in storage, so the best way to get hold of them is to grow your own. Research shows female flowers are by far the best, with a much higher overall polyphenol content than the smaller male blooms.

- **Skin deep** The highest concentrations of carotenoids are found in the skin of the courgette, which contains a huge 22 times more than the flesh.

- **Cooks' tips** Microwaving and frying courgettes in oil has been shown to increase levels of polyphenols and flavonoids in the fruits, while pressure cooking is the best way to enhance their antioxidant activity.

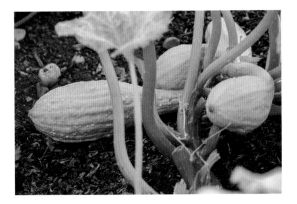

These unusual crookneck squashes have a delicious nutty flavour and will add diversity to your diet.

- **Storage** The fruits' antioxidant activity decreases significantly in storage. A study of 25 different vegetables found antioxidant levels decrease more in courgettes than in other vegetables – after seven days, over 30 per cent were lost.

Health benefits

Courgettes are a good source of fibre, vitamins B, C and K, and minerals, such as potassium and manganese. They are also rich in carotenoids, such as beta-carotene and lutein, which is important for eye health. Their lutein levels outstrip those found in other vegetables and a daily dose of 6mg reduces the risk of macular degeneration (an age-related eye disease) by 43 per cent. This equates to eating 7kg/15lb 7oz of tomatoes, 1kg/2lb 3oz of sweetcorn, or just 375g/13oz of courgettes.

Pumpkins & winter squashes

(includes *Cucurbita maxima, C. moschata & C. pepo*)

GROWING FOR GUT HEALTH

- **Go for orange** The colour of the flesh of winter squashes correlates to the type and level of carotenoids they contain. Squashes with bright orange flesh have a high carotene content, while yellow-fleshed pumpkins are rich in lutein. The best choices are the bright orange onion-type squashes, such as 'Hokkaido II', which have been found in studies to contain the highest levels of carotenoids.

- **Sow in spring** Sow seed indoors in late spring – sow two per 9cm/3½in pot and thin to the strongest seedling. Plant outside in full sun and free-draining soil when all risk of frost has passed. Leave at least 1m/3ft between these large sprawling plants. If they succumb to powdery mildew in hot, dry summers, remove affected leaves when you notice signs of damage to limit the spread of this fungal disease.

- **Select feed with care** To enhance their nutritional value, avoid using nitrogen fertilizers on your crops. Applying nitrogen can cause an incredible 70 per cent decrease in the polyphenol content of the fruits. However, using a potassium-rich fertilizer, such as seaweed extract, can increase the levels of carotenes in the fruits.

- **Give them heat** Growing pumpkins and squashes in areas with warmer temperatures causes an increase in carotenoids, so in hot summers, the fruits are likely to be richer in this polyphenol. Growing plants in a warm, sheltered spot, or even on a warm compost heap, will mimic these conditions and optimize their health value.

- **Harvesting and storage** The polyphenol content of pumpkins decreases as the fruits mature because they protect the crop from early deterioration and being eaten, allowing time for the seeds to develop. However, the carotenoid content increases as the fruit ripens, and continues to rise once it is harvested and put aside for storage. One study analyzing the nutritional qualities of pumpkins found an amazing 11 times more carotenoids in the crops after 12 weeks in storage.

- **Skin facts** The highest levels of carotenoids are found in the skins of squashes and pumpkins, so try roasting them, skin and all, for a delicious dish.

- **Prepare with oil** Boiling or steaming pumpkins retains more carotenoids than baking, while preparing your vegetables with oil makes these phytochemicals easier for the body to absorb.

Health benefits

Pumpkins and winter squashes are excellent sources of carotenoids, especially beta-carotene and, to a lesser extent, lycopene (also found in tomatoes) and alpha-carotene. They also contain lutein, which is good for eye health. Beta- and alpha-carotene both convert to vitamin A in the body, which is essential for human development and growth. Carotenoids, which give the flesh and flowers of pumpkins and winter squashes their characteristic yellow, orange or red colours, have high levels of antioxidant activity, and offer protection from heart disease and some cancers, such as skin and prostate cancer. The flesh also contains pectin, a type of prebiotic fibre that is good for our gut bacteria.

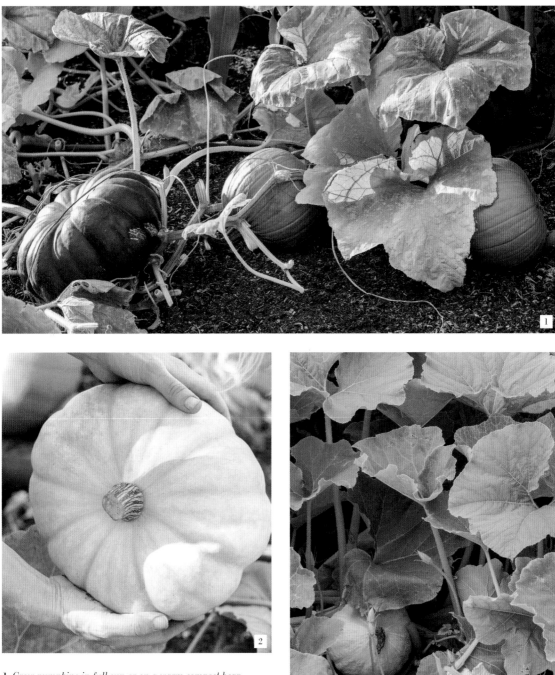

1. *Grow pumpkins in full sun or on a warm compost heap to increase their carotenoid content.* **2.** *Squash 'Crown Prince' has an excellent flavour and its bright orange flesh indicates its high carotene content.* **3.** *Onion-type squashes, such as this 'Uchiki Kuri' variety, have an extremely high carotenoid content.*

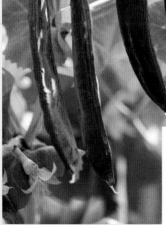
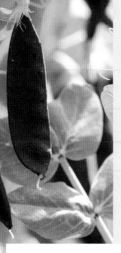
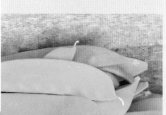

"Grow a variety
of colourful peas,
mangetout and
French beans for
good gut health."

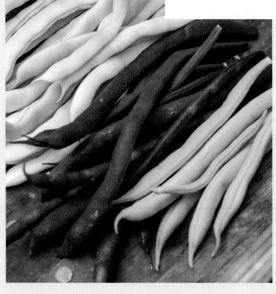
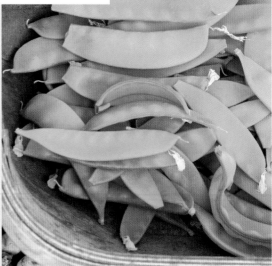

The legume family

Growing an assortment of peas and beans will provide you with tasty, protein-packed crops that can be added to a wide range of dishes. Some are not frost-hardy and climbers require support, but your efforts will be rewarded with crops rich in fibre and phytochemicals that store well.

A recent report published by the UN recommends that we all shift towards more plant-based diets to reduce our impact on the planet, which would especially help to reduce greenhouse gas emissions. Plants in the legume family are an excellent alternative source of protein to meat. The most popular are peas and beans and these powerhouses of nutrition offer a range of health benefits: as well as being low in fat, they are rich sources of folate, zinc, magnesium, iron and phytochemicals.

In addition, legumes are amazing foods to grow for gut health. The seed coats contain dietary fibre and phytochemicals that help to protect them from being eaten by insects or animals. The seeds themselves also offer high levels of resistant starch and fibre, which our gut microbes ferment and break down, helping to prevent inflammation, cardiovascular diseases and cancer of the colon. Compared to other vegetables we can grow in temperate climates, legumes offer the best sources of resistant starch, so including a mix of peas and beans in your edible garden provides our gut microbes with plenty of fuel.

The important phytochemicals in legumes include phenolic acids, flavonoids, such as quercetin and kaempferol, and saponin, which have anti-cancer effects and help to reduce cholesterol. Grow a range of different types, if you can, including some that can be dried and stored in winter for a continuous supply. Be adventurous with your varieties, as more diversity will provide your microbiota with different forms of starch and phytochemicals (see pages 16–21).

Health-boosting colours

The colour of a legume has a direct relationship with the level of phytochemicals, especially polyphenols, that they contain. A number of studies agree that darker red, bronze and black beans have a much higher phenolic content than paler green, yellow and white types. Black beans have the highest polyphenols content overall, followed by red, Great Northern (large white beans), pinto (mottled pink), navy beans (small white beans) and lastly, green beans.

Dark coloured beans have the highest levels of anthocyanins (see pages 20–21). They are present in purple-podded varieties of French bean, mangetout and pea. Mottled pink and yellow pigments on the seed coats are often due to the presence of tannins, which help increase immunity and lower blood pressure.

Clockwise from top left *Choose a range of colourful peas and beans, such as mangetout 'Shiraz'; mangetout 'Golden Sweet'; French beans 'Neckargold', 'Purple Teepee' and 'Tendergreen'; and mangetout 'Oregon Sugar Pod'.*

Peas & beans

(Pisum sativum, Vicia faba, Phaseolus vulgaris & Phaseolus coccineus)

GROWING FOR GUT HEALTH

• **Planting peas** Peas are quite hardy and germinate at relatively low temperatures. Sow five seeds per 9cm/3½in pot indoors in early spring and plant out these groups of seedlings once established at approximately 20cm/8in spacings. You can also sow directly in the ground in mid-spring, spacing seed approximately 5cm/2in apart. To support these climbing plants, I use natural pea sticks made of hazel branches, but you can also make a framework with netting. I often make a second sowing of peas

Healthy soya and lupins

Both lupins and soya beans are outstanding legumes to grow from a phytochemical perspective. Lupins are rich in a phytochemical called phytosterol, which has exceptional cholesterol-lowering properties. The most convenient way to grow them is to sprout the seeds (see pages 152–53).

Soya beans are particularly notable for their super-high isoflavones content, which promotes a healthy heart and bones. They also have a higher content of the phytochemical, tocopherols, than other legumes. This is a form of vitamin E, which is essential for healthy skin and protects the body from cancer and inflammation. Soya beans are easy to grow, but need a long, hot summer to do well. Sow them in pots indoors in late spring or early summer, and plant them out after the frosts, leaving 15cm/6in between the plants.

in late spring, which extends the harvesting period from late summer to early autumn. This second sowing is usually not as prolific as the first but still offers a useful harvest.

• **Sowing broad beans** Sow indoors or directly in the ground in autumn or early spring. I sow two seeds per 9cm/3½in pot and thin to the strongest seedling. Plant outside after the frosts at a spacing of 23cm/9in. To deter aphids, pinch out the growing tips when pods begin to set. Tall varieties, in particular, will need some support to grow: I use canes and strong twine to support the plants.

• **Growing French and runner beans** Sow directly into the ground or indoors in pots from late spring to early summer (following the advice for broad beans). Both French and runner beans are quite tender, so sow or plant them after the frosts at a spacing of 30–35cm/12–14in. French beans can either be dwarf types that require no support, or climbers, like runner beans, which both need a framework of canes to scramble up. Set beans sown under cover outside during the day and then bring them in again at night for a few weeks before planting outside.

• **Add stress** Growing peas and beans under conditions of mild stress will increase their polyphenol and carotenoid levels, as the plants' natural defence mechanisms go into action. Lower temperatures (but not frosty conditions) encourage the proliferation of polyphenols, while higher temperatures and light levels increase the carotenoid content and certain polyphenols, such as anthocyanins (see pages 20–21).

• **Aphids are your friends** Maybe not quite, but one interesting study into polyphenol levels in pea plants infested by aphids found higher levels

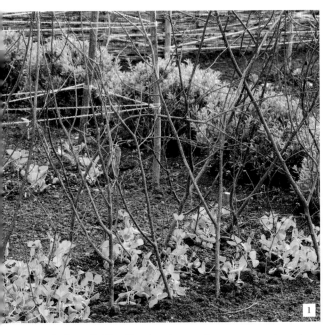

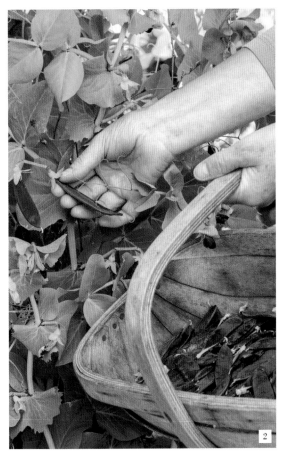

1. *Grow climbing French and runner beans up supports, such as sticks made from hazel branches.* 2. *Purple-podded mangetout 'Shiraz' is high in anthocyanins, which protect against cancer.*

of some phytochemicals, such as quercetin and apigenin, which help to protect plants from attack. So don't worry if you see a few aphids on your peas and avoid chemical pesticides. If you have a heavy infestation, remove aphids by hand (squish them) or use an organic soap spray, but remember that a few insects on your plants are good for your health, and they also maintain the garden's ecological balance.

- **Super sprouts** Germination of legumes has a dramatic effect on the phenolic content. It depends on the variety of legume being germinated but generally there is a leap in polyphenols. A recent Japanese study of popular legumes found that as seeds germinated there was at least a two-fold increase in polyphenol levels. (See pages 152–53 for tips on sprouting seeds at home.)

- **Keep their coats on** Some people peel beans, especially broad beans. The seed coats of peas and beans (the testa), contain the majority of the polyphenols, especially anthocyanins and tannins,

so it is really worth keeping them on for added nutrition. Their bitter edge adds another level to their flavour profile too.

- **Eat the pods** Pea pods are a good source of fibre and phytochemicals. Mangetout and sugar snaps can obviously be eaten raw, and the tougher pods of garden peas can be used in soups and stews.

- **Cooking effects** Legumes have the most resistant starch (see page 16–19) when eaten raw. If you cook them, they lose a significant amount, but this is regained if they are allowed to cool. Even reheated, they still have about 30 per cent more resistant starch than those cooked from fresh. Fructans, on the other hand, will leach into the water when beans and peas are boiled, so try steaming them instead.

Sweetcorn

(*Zea mays*)

Sweet, succulent, and a favourite among children, sweetcorn is well worth including in your productive plot. It is beneficial to our gut health and offers protection against eye and heart disease, Type 2 diabetes, and some forms of cancer.

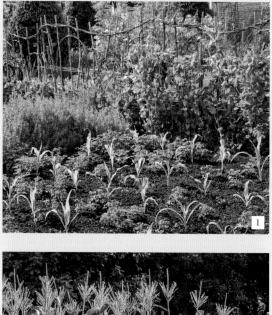

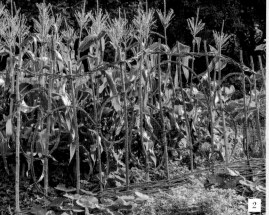

GROWING FOR GUT HEALTH

- **The brights have it** The varieties of corn we buy in the supermarkets are usually touted as being 'supersweet'. Often pale yellow in colour, or occasionally white, this corn is indeed sweeter, but at the expense of the nutritional value. Choose the brightest yellow varieties to grow at home and you will provide your microbes with the optimal amounts of carotenoids, namely beta-carotene, lutein and zeaxanthin, which together help to protect against eye disease, cancer and cardiovascular diseases. Yellow varieties contain nearly seven times the amount of beta-carotene and a startling 70 times more lutein than pale corn. Red, purple and blue corn are also excellent choices. Frequently just grown for their ornamental value, these brightly coloured varieties have a high anthocyanin content (see pages 20–21).

- **Growing and sowing** Sow two seeds per 9cm/ 3½in pot inside in late spring, or outside in the ground in late spring or early summer at a distance of 45cm/18in, again sowing two at each point. Thin to the strongest seedling. Sweetcorn

1. *Sweetcorn planted between oca* (Oxalis tuberosa) *utilizes space efficiently in small gardens.* 2. *Pick sweetcorn when it is fully ripe to maximize its carotenoid levels.* 3. *Bright yellow varieties of corn, or colourful red, blue or purple types, are much better nutritionally than pale, sweet cultivars.*

Health benefits

Sweetcorn is a good all-rounder vegetable for gut health. Not only does it provide a range of important phytochemicals, it's also a great source of resistant starch – that fermentable comfort food for your microbes (see pages 16–19). Corn is high in fibre, vitamins A, B, E and K, and minerals such as potassium, magnesium and phosphorus. Its polyphenols also give it more antioxidant activity than other common grains, including rice, oats or wheat. The health benefits include a healthy digestive system and a reduced risk of cardiovascular disease, Type 2 diabetes and some forms of cancer.

is wind pollinated so it is best to grow the plants close together in a grid formation to increase the likelihood of pollination occurring. As sweetcorn grows vertically, there is space available underneath to plant a secondary crop. Traditionally, trailing squashes (see pages 82–85) are grown with sweetcorn, and left to scramble in between the plants, but for the last few years I've been growing oca (*Oxalis tuberosa*), a delicious South American vegetable that tastes rather like a lemony potato.

- **Opt for a sunny spot** Polyphenol levels, especially anthocyanins, will be higher if you subject your sweetcorn to some stress. Plant in full sun to increase the UV light. Differences between night and day temperatures also have a positive effect on polyphenol levels, so plant in an exposed spot with supports to protect your crop from wind damage.

- **Be patient** Wait until the cobs are fully ripened before picking, since their carotenoid and polyphenol content increases until maturity. In fact, if you leave the corn to dry on the cob the polyphenol level is even higher – dry corn has a delicious nutty flavour. and can be stored and added to cooked dishes.

- **Sprout seeds in sunlight** Sprouting sweetcorn seed (the corn kernels) increases the level of polyphenols by over seven times. Leave corn to dry on the cob to save the seed for sprouting, and allow it to germinate in sunlight, rather than in the dark, for the highest nutrient value.

- **Avoid refined corn products** About 87 per cent of the polyphenols in sweetcorn are found in the bran (the outer layer of each kernel) and the germ (the sweet, bright yellow nugget on the inside, at the base of the kernel). In corn products, such as refined corn oil, these parts are often removed, leaving very little nutritional value. Growing your own sweetcorn to eat straight from the cob helps you to gain as much of the fibre and polyphenols as possible.

- **Fuel for microbes** While corn is at its sweetest when eaten fresh from the plant, after a day or so the sucrose starts to convert to starch, which is very useful to your microbes. If you can, keep some of the cobs you harvest in the refrigerator for a few days to give your gut microbes beneficial starchy fuel to ferment and digest.

- **Heat for more treats** Boiling sweetcorn in the traditional way causes phytochemicals to be leached out into the cooking water. Try microwaving or steaming the cobs instead to retain the nutrients. The process of heating sweetcorn during cooking has actually been found to increase antioxidant and polyphenol levels too.

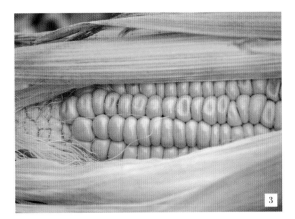

The potato family

Potatoes are a staple ingredient for many delicious dishes, and this versatile crop has much more to offer in terms of health benefits than is widely believed. The potato family also includes other highly nutritious vegetables, such as tomatoes, aubergines and peppers.

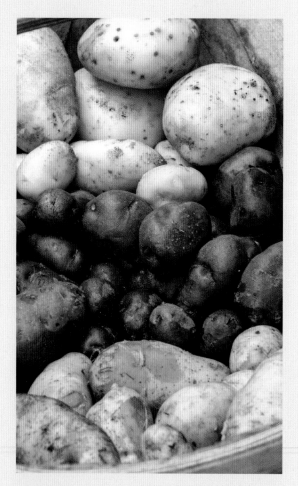

Purple potatoes, such as 'Purple Majesty' and 'Salad Blue', contain the highest levels of polyphenols.

"Rich in the fibre that fuels our gut microbes, potatoes are also an excellent source of vitamin C and phytochemicals."

The potato family is a broad church and includes very familiar and some more unusual vegetables and fruit. Potatoes, aubergines, tomatoes, chillies and peppers are all members and each offers a range of health benefits for the home-grower. Slightly more unusual crops, such as tomatillos and cape gooseberries, also belong to this group. As there is so much diversity within the potato family, I have detailed the specific benefits of each and how to grow them in the pages that follow.

Potatoes
(Solanum tuberosum)

GROWING FOR GUT HEALTH

- **Select a rainbow** Colourful purple potatoes take a bit of getting used to, but they are worth growing because they have a much higher polyphenol content than their pale relatives. Purple ranks the highest, followed by red, yellow and white cultivars – purple potatoes have almost four times as much as other varieties. They are also very rich sources of anthocyanins (see pages 20–21) and have a similar level to berries, such as cranberries and blueberries. There are a number of different cultivars to choose from, but the best are purple inside and out, such as 'Purple Majesty', 'All Blue' or 'Vitelotte'. Try other types, too, for their health benefits. Yellow cultivars, for example, have high levels of lutein, with up to ten times the carotenoids, which are associated with good eye health and a strong immune system, of their white cousins.

- **Planting first and second earlies** Plant tubers directly in the ground in mid-spring, approximately 30–40cm/12–16in apart. Pile soil up around the stems as they emerge (a technique known as 'earthing up') until the risk of frost has passed. Harvest this crop in early summer.

- **Main-crop planting** Plant tubers directly in the ground in late spring, again earthing up the stems as they grow while there is a risk of frost damage. Harvest this later crop in midsummer.

- **Babies are best** Studies show that baby or immature potatoes contain higher amounts of phytochemicals than mature tubers, so it's worth harvesting them on the small size for optimal nutritional benefit. Small new potatoes also have up to twice as much vitamin C.

Health benefits

The popular belief that potatoes have no nutritional value is simply not true. They are high in fibre, especially in the skin – one medium-sized potato provides over ten per cent of your recommended daily intake. The fibre and resistant starch they contain helps to lower blood glucose levels, protect the lining of the gut and promote good digestion. Potatoes are also a great source of vitamins C and B, folate and potassium, which is essential for muscle and nerve functioning. They also contain beta-carotene and polyphenols (see pages 20–21).

- **Keep them cool** Anthocyanin levels and total polyphenol content increases at lower temperatures so avoid growing potatoes in very sheltered and warm spots. For example, do not grow them next to a sunny wall that will trap heat.

- **Wait before eating** Although potatoes are delicious fresh, most studies show their polyphenol levels increase after storage, allowing us to store them into winter without compromising the health benefits.

- **Cook and cool** Resistant starch in potatoes is influenced by cooking them. Most studies find cooked and chilled potatoes have more than hot or raw potatoes (the latter are toxic). The process of cooking disrupts the structure of the starch molecules in the tubers, but, when cooled, these molecules reform into resistant starch, which remains high even when they are reheated.

Tomatoes
(Solanum lycopersicum)

GROWING FOR GUT HEALTH

- **Choose a cherry** Cherries tomatoes have higher levels of beta-carotene, flavonoids and vitamin C compared to traditional large-fruited varieties. In fact, they have at least twice the amount of flavonoids than the bigger fruits, so if you have limited space, plump for a cherry type.

- **Experiment with colour** Diversity is key. Grow and eat different-coloured tomatoes to benefit from the different types of phytochemical. Red varieties have the highest amount of lycopene and beta-carotene. Orange types have the greatest concentration of vitamin E, while yellow fruits have the most polyphenols. Different varieties of tomato contain specific phytochemicals in varying quantities.

- **Start sowing early** Tomatoes can be sown in early spring in pots or modules indoors. Either grow on under cover or plant outside in late spring to early summer, once the risk of frost has passed.

- **Keep on the dry side** Stressing tomato plants by giving them less water will enhance their phytochemical levels and antioxidant activity, according to a Mediterranean study. Too much water can lead to the deterioration of the phytochemicals, especially if the fruits split. Try to balance watering crops to ensure a decent yield, and keeping them on the dry side to enhance their nutritional value and flavour.

- **Expose to the elements** Tomatoes grown outside are subjected to more environmental stress. The bigger difference between night and day temperatures and exposure to more sunlight result in plants producing more defensive phytochemicals. However, tomatoes are not hardy plants and need

Health benefits

People used to be afraid of eating tomatoes, probably because they are related to the highly toxic plant, deadly nightshade. Their botanical name, *Solanum lycopersicum,* means the 'wolf peach', revealing just how wary people were. I'm so glad we're over that now because tomatoes are packed with nutrients. Rich sources of vitamin C and folate, and minerals such as potassium, tomatoes also contain carotenoids, including lycopene and beta-carotene, which converts to vitamin A in the body. Scientific studies have shown that lycopene helps to prevent cancer, especially prostate cancer, and protects against heart disease. Tomatoes also have high levels of antioxidant activity and polyphenols, including flavonoids (see pages 20–21).

warm temperatures for the fruit to mature, so plant them in full sun in a relatively sheltered spot.

- **Allow the colour to develop** The lycopene content of red tomatoes increases significantly as the fruits mature – levels peak when they are completely red.

- **Optimum temperatures** Temperature has a significant impact on the polyphenol levels in tomatoes. Lycopene is highly sensitive to extreme temperatures – its production is very limited below 12°C/54°F and stops completely at 32°C/90°F and above. In a hot summer, provide your plants with shade netting to lessen the detrimental effects on lycopene production.

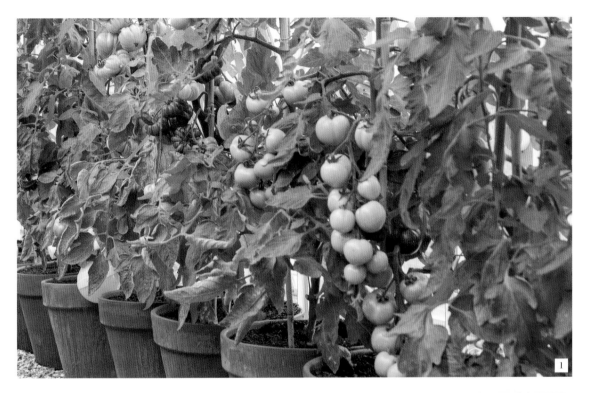

- **Ripen off the vine** A study of tomato 'Moneymaker', comparing the fruits when vine-ripened and ripened post-harvest, found that the latter were higher in phytochemicals. So, pick tomatoes when under-ripe, and allow them to ripen at room temperature.

- **Cook for health** Lycopene is more abundant and available for the body to absorb in cooked tomatoes. This is because raw fruits are over 95 per cent water, which is lost while cooking, making the lycopene more concentrated in purées and sauces. Cooking also changes the chemical structure of lycopene, making it easier for the body to absorb.

- **Salt stress** The tomatoes on plants subjected to salt stress have 35–85 per cent more lycopene. Salt also causes fruit to ripen more quickly. To try this at home, dilute one tablespoon of sea salt in 8 litres/ 14 pints of water (a standard watering can) and give your plants a soil drench. Only do this a few times throughout the growing season, or salt will build up in the soil and reduce the yield.

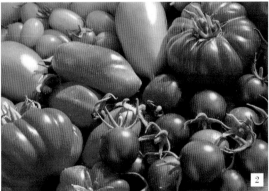

1. Outdoor tomatoes are subjected to more stress, which increases their phytochemical content, than crops grown in a glasshouse.
2. Grow a diverse range of different-coloured tomatoes for a wider variety of health-boosting phytochemicals.

Aubergines (eggplants)
(*Solanum melongena*)

GROWING FOR GUT HEALTH

• **Pick a colour** There are three different types of aubergine, botanically speaking: the egg-shaped varieties, long and slender types, and dwarf fruits. They also come in a wide range of colours, from the dark purple fruit everyone is familiar with, through to green, pink, white, stripy and mottled types. Generally, the darker the skin of the fruit, the higher the level of anthocyanins (see pages 20–21). However, apart from this, there doesn't seem to be a strong correlation between colour and total polyphenol content, so take your pick.

• **Cultivars count** There is a significant variation in polyphenol content between different cultivars of aubergine, according to a US study that looked at the levels in seven cultivars grown commercially. It found aubergine 'Black Magic' had nearly three times as much antioxidant polyphenols as other varieties, so look out for it in seed catalogues.

• **Wild relatives** If you can find the seed of natural species of aubergine, a study from India (home of the aubergine) shows that they have significantly higher polyphenol content than the cultivars. *Solanum sisymbriifolium*, *Solanum torvum* and *Solanum incanum* are all recommended species. Landraces (varieties local to a specific geographical area) of aubergine have also been found to have higher levels of polyphenols than cultivars.

• **Sow indoors** Sow seed indoors in early spring in pots or modules. Place in a propagator or on a warm windowsill as seed needs 20–30°C/68–86°F to germinate. Do not plant outside until after the frosts, and space plants 45cm/18in apart. Plants may need to be staked during the growing season, especially varieties with large fruits. Prevent spider

mite, which sometimes attacks indoor-grown aubergine plants, by increasing humidity levels or use the predatory mites *Phytoseiulus persimilis* as a biological control.

• **Grow outside** The polyphenol content of aubergines has been found in studies to decrease in high temperatures, so grow your aubergines outside, where possible, which will expose them to colder night-time temperatures.

• **Little treats** Small-fruited varieties, especially those with purple skins, have higher levels of antioxidant activity and polyphenol content. As supermarket fruits are often large, this is another good reason to grow your own at home.

• **Storage tip** The polyphenol content of aubergine stored for up to three days in refrigerated conditions actually goes up but then declines thereafter. Keep your fruit in the refrigerator for a few days before eating it for the maximum health benefits.

• **Leave the skin on** Do not remove the skins of aubergines when cooking, as they are very high in flavonoids, especially anthocyanins.

• **Cut and cook** You've probably noticed the flesh of aubergines turns brown once the fruit is cut. This is due to the phenolic compounds being exposed to the air and oxidizing, which provides a good indicator of the high phytochemical content. When cutting, use a sharp, thin knife to minimize any damage to the aubergine fruits and losses in phytochemicals. As phytochemicals can also be leached when cooking in oil or water, try to add the residue liquids to the meal, or include them in sauces or soups, for example, to make sure you retain as many of the health benefits as possible.

Health benefits

Often thought of as a Mediterranean vegetable, aubergines actually originate from India, China and Japan, and have gradually spread to the West. They are ranked as one of the top ten vegetables for antioxidant activity, due to their very high phytochemical content. The skin contains a specific type of anthocyanin called nasunin, which gives the fruit its characteristic deep purple colour. A powerful antioxidant, nasunin protects brain cells from free-radical damage, thereby maintaining our cognitive skills. Aubergines are also high in fibre, B vitamins, potassium and other phytochemicals, such as carotenoids (see pages 20–21) and tannins, which help with blood clotting and reduce blood pressure. The pulp is also rich in phenolic acid, especially chlorogenic acid, which has excellent anti-cancer and anti-inflammatory properties and protects against diabetes.

1. Choose varieties with small fruits, and dark purple skin for greater antioxidant activity. 2. If you have space, grow more than one type of aubergine to increase diversity in your diet.

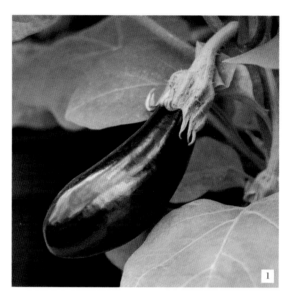

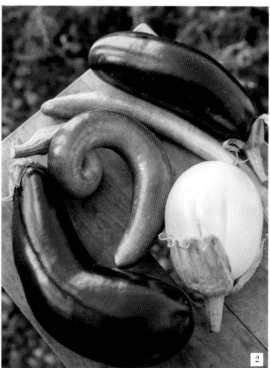

Chillies & peppers
(Capsicum frutescens and *C. annuum)*

GROWING FOR GUT HEALTH

- **Start in spring** Sow seed indoors in pots or modules in a warm environment in early spring. Chillies can then be grown on indoors or outdoors in a sheltered, sunny spot. If planting outside, wait until any risk of frost has passed, and space plants approximately 40–50cm/16–20in apart.

- **Keep colour in mind** The fruits of pepper and chilli plants tend to change colour over the growing season as they mature, usually developing from green or white to orange and red. Orange and red peppers contain the highest levels of beta-carotene and a specific carotenoid called capsanthin, which gives the peppers and chillies their characteristic red colour. Capsanthin is an antioxidant that has been found to help protect against cancer of the colon, among other health benefits. Red peppers and chillies are also a great source of lycopene, more usually found in tomatoes (see page 94).

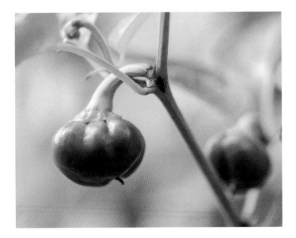

Harvest your chillies as they change colour throughout the growing season, to benefit from the different phytochemical changes that happen in the fruits as they mature.

Green peppers contain the highest levels of carotenoids, such as lutein, and polyphenols (see pages 20–21). Harvest your peppers and chillies over the growing season, ensuring you eat a range of different-coloured fruits, and consequently a diverse range of different phytochemicals.

Health benefits

Chillies and peppers are generally eaten in small quantities because of their heat, but they still offer many health benefits. They are high in vitamins B6, C, and K, and have among the highest levels of antioxidants of any vegetable.

The hottest chilli in the world is called 'Carolina Reaper' – it is 200 times hotter than a jalapeño. Although incredibly high in antioxidants, it's virtually inedible for all but the boldest of chilli eaters, such as the man who ate 22 of them in 60 seconds and holds the Guinness World Record for the hottest-chilli-eating contest. The main compound in chillies that gives them their heat is capsaicin, which helps to protect against cancer and diseases such as diabetes. It also helps to relieve pain. Capsaicin is a powerful phytochemical that has evolved to protect the fruits from being eaten. It triggers pain signals in the nerves, causing a stringent burning sensation, while not causing any actual physical injury. However, capsaicin does not affect birds, allowing them to eat the fruit and disperse the seeds.

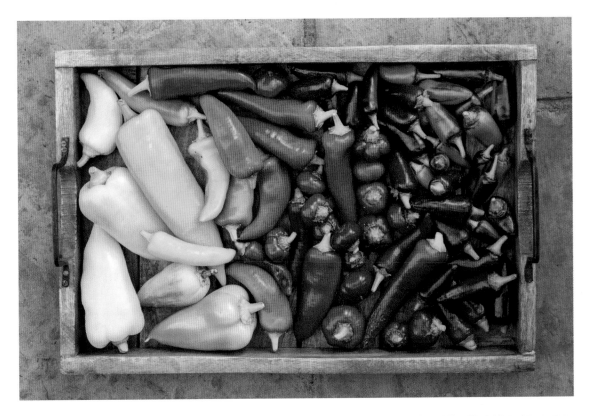

The hotter the chilli, the higher the levels of capsaicin, which is a powerful phytochemical that protects against cancer and diabetes, and helps to relieve pain.

• **Good storage** As with many other types of fruit and vegetable, the polyphenols in chillies and peppers increases slightly over time. Try eating some of yours fresh, but also store some in the refrigerator for even greater nutritional value. Fermenting them often increases polyphenol levels even further (see page 176 for my favourite fiery chilli sauce fermentation recipe).

• **Steam, roast or fry** Uncooked peppers and chillies have the highest phytochemical content, while boiling and freezing leads to a reduction in their health value. Steaming, roasting and stir-frying are the best ways to cook these vegetables to benefit the most from their antioxidant properties.

Heat is for better health

There is a direct correlation between the heat of chilli peppers and the levels of capsaicin. Heat in chillies is measured in SHU (Scoville Heat Units). One study showed the superhot habanero-type chilli pepper (*Capsicum chinense*) with a 320,000 SHU had 1,000 times the capsaicin levels of a mild red chilli with 3,200 SHU. So the hotter the better when it comes to the nutritional value of your chilli peppers.

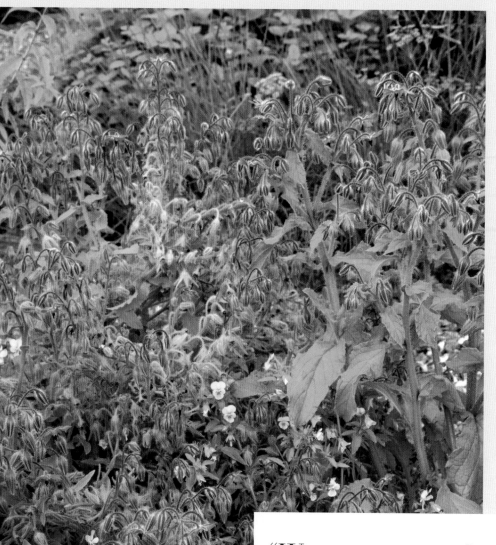

"We may not eat herbs in large amounts, but they are still very nutritious because their phytochemical content is so high."

Herbs

With hundreds of herbs to choose from, all containing very high levels of health-promoting phytochemicals, these easy-to-grow plants offer the perfect way to include more crop varieties in your vegetable garden, while increasing the rich diversity in your diet.

Herbs include members of many different plant groups, such as the mint, carrot and verbena families. Many are prized for their exceptionally high phytochemical content, often revealed by their strong, aromatic scents when the leaves are crushed.

The polyphenols in herbs and spices help to protect the plants against pests and diseases, the damaging effects of sunlight and from being eaten by pests. Many contain fantastically high levels of these beneficial compounds compared to other edible plants; for example, dried peppermint has about 120 times more polyphenols than red wine. However, these compounds in herbs and spices can be difficult to digest, and we need the assistance of our gut microbes to absorb them and access the health benefits, which include protection against cancer, cardiovascular disease, inflammatory bowel syndrome (IBS), and Alzheimer's disease.

Although we don't eat large amounts of herbs, they offer a great way to increase diversity in our diets and are very beneficial because their phytochemical content is so high. For ways to include more herbs in your meals, look to Asian and Mediterranean cuisines, where they are used in abundance.

Most herbs are very easy to grow in the garden or in pots on a patio or windowsill, but the types we grow, the parts of the plant we harvest and how we choose to grow them all have a significant impact on their phytochemical profiles.

Health benefits

There's a plethora of herb varieties to grow and including a diversity of different types will ensure you gain from as many different types of polyphenols as possible. The US Dietary Association (USDA) has produced a report listing the top 100 foods by polyphenol content (see pages 20–21) and many high-ranking types were herbs and spices. The top ten are shown in the table below. It's not an exhaustive list and some of my favourites, such as turmeric, perilla and chervil, are not on it but well worth growing.

POLYPHENOL CONTENT OF TEN HERBS AND SPICES

HERB / SPICE	VALUE IN MG PER 100G/3.5OZ
Cloves	15,188mg/0.5oz
Peppermint (dried)	11,960mg/0.4oz
Oregano (dried)	2,319mg/0.08oz
Celery seed	2,094mg/0.07oz
Sage (dried)	1,207mg/0.05oz
Rosemary (dried)	1,018mg/0.04oz
Spearmint (dried)	956mg/0.035oz
Thyme (dried)	878mg/0.03oz
Basil (dried)	322mg/0.01oz
Ginger (dried)	202mg/0.007oz

GROWING FOR GUT HEALTH

- **Mimic native conditions** There are lots of different types of herb so it is difficult to give general growing advice, but if you look at the habitats your chosen varieties have come from, you can aim to emulate those conditions. Many common herbs, such as sage, thyme, basil and rosemary, are from the Mediterranean region, which experiences hot, dry summers. Consequently, these herbs need full sun and free-draining growing media or soil. If you have shadier conditions and moist soil, opt for mint, lemon balm, chives, parsley and chervil.

- **Hold the water** Several studies have shown that water stress increases the polyphenol content of herbs, although some are more tolerant of drought than others. To create the optimum growing conditions, plant your herbs in free-draining soil, or a gritty compost mix if planting in pots. Minimize or avoid watering your plants to encourage them to accumulate as many phytochemicals as possible during the growing season.

- **Harvest before blooming** The optimal time to harvest the foliage in terms of polyphenol content is at the very start of the flowering period or when the plant is in full leaf. Once plants are in full bloom, the polyphenol production is concentrated mostly in the flowers and there's a big reduction in the leaves and stems. Keep picking your herbs to keep them at that optimum early-flowering stage for longer. However, remember that the flowers and seeds of many herbs are also edible and offer an excellent source of polyphenols to include in your recipes.

- **Afternoon picking** The best time of day to pick your herbs is around the middle of the afternoon. This is because sunlight is needed for the biochemical reactions to take place to create the phytochemicals in the leaves. Strong sunlight also causes plants stress, which means that herbs are likely to produce more of these defensive compounds in the afternoon to protect themselves from the damaging rays.

- **Leave to dry** Drying herbs significantly increases the polyphenol content of the plants. Studies show that in many cases dried herbs have at least three to four times the amount of polyphenols found in fresh leaves. For example, dried dill contains six times more polyphenols than fresh, and dried sage and coriander both contain nearly 16 times more than their fresh counterparts. This is thought to be because enzymes present in plants, which cause the deterioration of polyphenols, break down during the drying process.

Regional variations

The chemical composition of herbs can vary considerably depending on where they were grown in the world. Plants evolve differently, even within species, according to the local environment and growing conditions they experience. Studies of turmeric plants from different parts of Thailand, for instance, showed their levels of curcumin varied widely – curcumin is a phytochemical with very promising health benefits. Similarly, thyme from different parts of the world contains very different types and quantities of phytochemicals. For example, thymol, a potent antioxidant that can help to protect us against respiratory and cardiovascular disorders, featured in essential-oil extracts from Estonian wild thyme, but researchers found no trace of it at all in samples from Lithuania. Thymol acts as an insecticide in the plant, so perhaps Lithuanian thyme is less at risk of pest attack.

While home-growers are not yet able to select herbs from different areas according to their phytochemical make-up, it is worth knowing that they have great genetic diversity. This is beneficial because the greater the genetic diversity, the more plants are able to adapt to future threats.

1. Like other members of the onion family, chives contain cholesterol-lowering alliin. 2. Perilla is an easy-to-grow herb with attractive dark leaves high in anthocyanins. 3. Rosemary is a rich source of polyphenols and has high antioxidant activity.

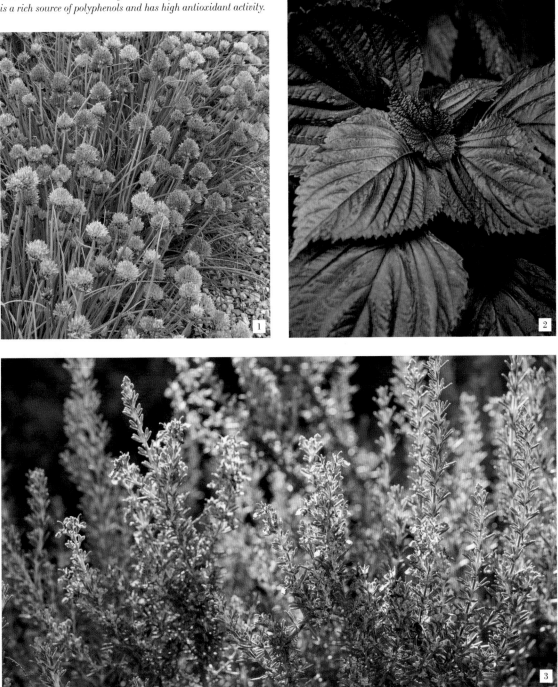

"Grow and eat your own freshly harvested organic apples for their incredible benefits to your gut microbes and health."

Apples

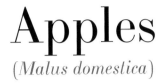

(Malus domestica)

Rich in prebiotic fibre, vitamins, minerals and phytochemicals, it seems that the old adage about an apple a day keeping the doctor away is based on facts, and growing your own fruit trees in the garden allows you to increase the health benefits even further.

We have always been told an apple a day keeps the doctor away, but why? Eating apples is beneficial to us, not just because of the vitamins and minerals they contain, but also because they are rich in the fibre that feeds our gut microbes. In addition, they contain phytochemicals, which vary according to the variety, the site and soil conditions in which the trees are growing, the season the fruits are harvested, and how they are stored and processed, all of which are more easily managed if you grow them at home. With all these benefits it is definitely worth planting a tree in your garden – or even a dwarf variety in a large container if your space is limited.

The walled garden I manage with my partner, David, used to be an old apple orchard and we are lucky to have two dozen old apple trees. These gorgeous, gnarled trees still produce a heavy crop most years and while we don't stand a chance of eating all the apples from them, in autumn we make juice with the excess, producing hundreds of bottles of delicious juice to enjoy through the year.

Health benefits

Apples contain pectin, a type of prebiotic dietary fibre that is fermented by bacteria in the gut to produce short-chain fatty acids (see pages 16–17). Recent studies have shown that pectin derived from apples increases the number and diversity of friendly flora in the gut, with health benefits that include a reduced risk of some cancers, heart disease and asthma.

Apples also contain phytochemicals, including phenolic acids, flavonoids and anthocyanins in red-skinned varieties (see pages 20–21) that may protect against Alzheimer's disease and diabetes, and help to maintain good bone health. Apples have excellent antioxidant activity too.

Research also shows that eating this combination of pectin and polyphenols in apples enhances their beneficial effects, proving that we need to eat wholefoods rather than processed products.

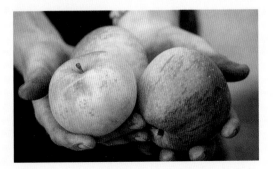

PLANTING AND PRUNING APPLES

Plant in autumn Trees can be purchased in two different forms: bare-root and container-grown. Bare-root trees can be planted when dormant, from late autumn until early spring, and container-grown trees can be planted at any time of the year, although I would always recommend planting any apple tree in late autumn. The trees then have time to establish root systems over winter, and will benefit from natural rainwater rather than needing extra irrigation. With climate change and more unpredictable springs in many areas, this practice is likely to become increasingly important. When planting, make sure your tree is planted at the same depth as it was in the nursery – you will see the darker soil mark on the stem – and ensure the rootstock union (bump on stem) is above the soil level.

Ideal rootstocks Apple trees are usually grafted on to rootstocks, which determine the size and vigour of the plant; the degree of cropping; pest and disease resistance; and the health of the root system. The most common types include:
• M27 – creates a very small plant and is often used for stepovers and dwarf bushes (height and spread: 1.8m/6ft).
• M9 – a dwarfing rootstock, often used for cordons (height and spread: 1.8–3m/6–10ft).
• M26 – makes a compact tree and is useful for small gardens and cordons (height and spread: 2.5–3.5m/8–12ft).
• MM106 – a semi-dwarfing rootstock that will produce a medium-sized tree suitable for larger gardens (height and spread: 3.5–5.5m/12–18ft).

Pollination partners A few types of apple are self-fertile, but most trees need more than one type of apple to ensure pollination occurs and the fruit sets. Choose at least two cultivars that flower at similar times of the year to enable cross-pollination. If you don't have space for

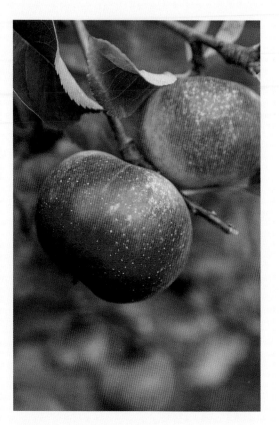

more than one tree, look around your local area for other apple trees or wild crab apples in the vicinity that can act as a pollination partner.

Pruning tips Pruning helps to ensure trees remain in good health and encourages more crops. Pruning is also beneficial from a nutritional perspective, since it helps to expose the fruits to more light, which increases their polyphenol levels. For an effective use of space, and to ensure the most light reaches the fruit, train trees from a young age against a wall or fence as cordons, fans or espaliers. Also use reflective mulches or pale gravel under the trees to reflect the light on to the lower branches.

GROWING FOR GUT HEALTH

• **Choosing varieties** A UK study analysed the polyphenol content of eight of the most popular apple varieties found in supermarkets. It found the richest sources were in 'Braeburn', followed in order by 'Red Delicious' (now known as 'Starking'), 'Cripps Pink' (formerly Pink Lady), 'Royal Gala', 'Granny Smith', bramley, 'Golden Delicious', and lastly 'Fuji', which had the lowest level.

Alternatively, opt for a local heritage variety, which research shows have higher levels of polyphenols than modern cultivars. A German study found old local apple cultivars have up to 30 per cent more polyphenols than new varieties, so 'going local' is good for nutrition and helps to support diversity in the gene pool. When it comes to dessert apples, red varieties, especially those with pink flesh, are generally best, as they are higher in anthocyanins (see pages 20–21). A number of studies also show cider apples, which have a much sourer flavour, have significantly higher polyphenol levels.

• **Wild crab apples** Studies have shown that wild crab apples have a higher phytochemical content and antioxidant activity than dessert apples, with red forms offering the highest value. A study of over 450 varieties of cultivated apples, and 29 species of wild apple (including crab apples) found that on average the wild fruits also have nearly twice the amount of vitamin C – some varieties have up to 26 times as much. There seems to also be a correlation between smaller fruits and higher vitamin content.

• **Family trees** If you want diversity in a small space you could try growing a 'family' apple tree. This has a number of different varieties of apples grafted on to one rootstock. They usually have three or four types of apple on one tree, but I have heard of one tree with 250 varieties. That's quite a mutant!

Eat the whole apple, core and all if you can, to absorb the most microbes from the fruit, which in turn may help to increase the beneficial microbes in our gut.

• **Teaming with microbes** A study has found that every apple contains on average 100 million micro-organisms. When we eat the fruit, we ingest these microbes and some of them may colonize our gut, increasing the diversity of good bacteria. This highlights the importance of growing fruit and vegetables organically, without using chemical pesticides that may harm the plant microbiota (see pages 26–27). Most microbes are found in the seeds and the core of the apple, so eat the whole fruit, raw and freshly picked, to maximize benefits.

• **Juicy facts** Fresh apple juice is an excellent way to process a glut of apples. By doing so, the fibre content of the apples is lost but significant quantities of phytochemicals are retained. Fresh juice made from cider apples has the highest phytochemical content, with up to six times the polyphenols of dessert apples. If you're buying apple juice, go for cloudy types, which have up to four times more polyphenols than clear juice.

• **Eat the peel** Rich in dietary fibre, apple peel has two to six times more polyphenols than the flesh, and red varieties also contain anthocyanins. The core has the next highest polyphenol content.

• **Store for more** Keeping apples in cool storage for up to four months actually increases the polyphenol levels, making them the perfect winter snack.

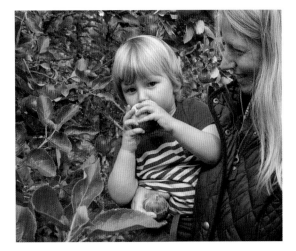

Pears

(*Pyrus communis*)

In China, pears are symbols of immortality, and they possess many excellent nutritional benefits. Rich in vitamins A and C, as well as a range of phytochemicals, few fruits have more fibre, making them the perfect fuel for our gut microbes.

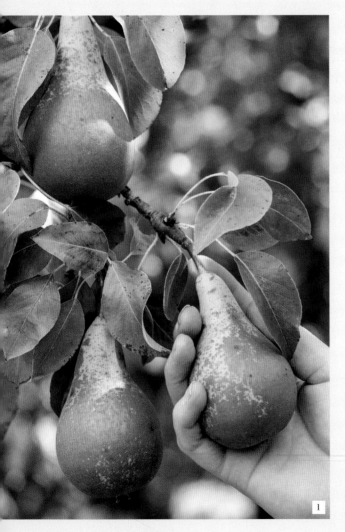

GROWING FOR GUT HEALTH

- **Choose red or green** When selecting pear varieties for the garden, choose red- and green-fruited varieties, as they have higher polyphenol levels than yellow fruits. Studies into commonly grown cultivars showed 'Forelle' had the highest polyphenol content, followed by 'Taylor's' (closely related to 'Doyenné du Comice'), 'Peckham's' and, lastly, 'Conference'.

- **Go local** Like the findings into apples, research shows polyphenols are higher in local pear varieties than standard cultivars. If you have time, research old varieties grown in your area and see if you can source a tree – it is also likely to be better suited to your local garden conditions.

- **Take stock** There are two standard rootstocks for pear trees. Quince C is a semi-dwarfing type, suitable for small trees of a height and spread of 2.5–5.5m/8–18ft, cordons and espaliers. Quince A is marginally more vigorous, suitable for larger trees and espaliers, with a height and spread of 3–6m/10–20ft.

- **Planting pear trees** Plant as bare-root trees or container-grown trees in the autumn. When planting,

1. *Pick your pears when ripe for the highest levels of the prebiotic fibre, pectin.* 2. *'Forelle' pears have a particularly high polyphenol content, according to recent research.*

Health benefits

Pears distinguish themselves nutritionally by being very good sources of fibre – one medium-sized pear contains nearly 25 per cent of the recommended daily intake. They are also packed with vitamins, especially vitamin A and C, and have high levels of carotenoids, which are critical for maintaining good eye sight as we age. Pears will also help you to top up your levels of flavonoids, including anthocyanins in the case of red pears, which have anti-cancer and anti-inflammatory effects, and help to decrease the risk of Type 2 diabetes.

make sure your tree is planted at the same depth as it was in its container or the nursery (look for the soil mark on the stem) and ensure the rootstock union is above the soil level.

• **Pollination partners** Most pear trees need a pollination partner in order to set fruit effectively. Ideally plant two different cultivars that flower at a similar time. If you don't have space for two, check to see if there is another suitable pear tree in a nearby garden.

• **Let in the light** In small spaces, train your trees as cordons or espaliers against a wall or fence. This ensures more light reaches the fruit, resulting in higher levels of polyphenols. Also use reflective mulches or pale gravel under the trees to reflect light on to the lower branches.

• **Do not peel** The peel of a pear is rich in flavonoids, especially anthocyanins in red varieties (see pages 20–21) and contains 17 times the amount of these cancer-fighting compounds than the flesh. In fact, if you remove the peel up to 25 per cent of the polyphenols can be lost, as well as significant amounts of dietary fibre. When compared to the flesh, the core of a pear also has the highest levels of chlorogenic acid, which may help to reduce blood pressure and regulate glucose and insulin levels, thereby protecting against Type 2 diabetes.

• **Harvest when ripe** A study into pears found that the pectin levels are highest when the flesh is soft, juicy and ripe. Pectin is amazing, fermentable fuel for gut bacteria. Test for ripeness by gently twisting each fruit upwards on the branch. If it falls away easily, it's ready. You can also cut into the pear and check the colour of the core and seeds, which are dark in colour compared to the flesh when ripe.

• **Cloudy goodness** Cloudy pear juice is much better for you than clear pear juice, as it contains more of the pulp and up to 40 per cent more phytochemicals. Make it from your own pears and include the pulp to guarantee its nutrient value.

• **Eat freshly picked** The vitamin C content of pears is reduced by 75 per cent after a week, so eat them fresh. To ensure the fruits retain a high polyphenol content and antioxidant activity, do not leave them to become overripe before picking – this can also result in the pears developing a mealy texture.

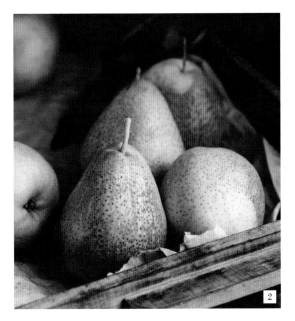

2

Peaches

(Prunus persica)

Growing your own peach tree against a sunny wall or on a boundary fence will provide you with rich pickings in summer. Research also shows that you can boost the fruits' phytochemical content even further by harvesting them at just the right time.

GROWING FOR GUT HEALTH

The botanical name for peach, *Prunus persica*, suggests that they originally came from Persia but the cultivated fruits are more likely to be from wild ancestors in China – 8,000-year-old peach stones have been found in Zhejiang Province in China.

- **Red is the winner** The French variety 'Pêche de Vigne', a blood peach, is considered to be one of the finest for flavour. It may also be among the best for health since red-fleshed peaches have over six times more polyphenols than white peaches, and nearly five times more than yellow varieties. Not all studies agree whether yellow- or white-fleshed peaches have more polyphenols, but yellow fruits are definitely a better source of carotenoids, with up to ten times as much as white-fleshed varieties.

Health benefits

Peaches are a great source of dietary fibre, vitamins A and C, and potassium. They also contain a range of phytochemicals, including polyphenols and carotenoids. These help to protect against some types of cancer, boost immunity and possibly reduce allergies by preventing the release of histamines.

- **Planting peaches** St Julien A is the most common rootstock, producing a peach tree with a height and spread of about 3.5m/12ft. Plant as a bare-root or container-grown tree in a sunny, sheltered spot in autumn at the same depth as it was in its pot or the nursery (look for the soil mark on the stem). Ensure the rootstock union is above the soil level.

- **Pollinate by hand** Peach trees tend not to need a pollination partner tree, but if you do not see many natural pollinators on the flowers, you may need to hand-pollinate them with a paintbrush.

- **Find a sunny spot** Peaches exposed to high levels of sunlight have more polyphenols, such as chlorogenic acid (see page 109) and anthocyanins (see pages 20–21). Train your tree into a fan or espalier against a wall or a fence and thin the fruits to allow more space and light around each peach. Also use reflective mulches made from natural materials, such as pale coloured stone or gravel, under the trees so that they bounce light on to the fruit on the lower branches.

- **Keep dry** Water stress increases the polyphenol levels and antioxidant activity in peaches, so avoid irrigating your trees unless it is absolutely necessary. The exception to this rule is when planting new fruit trees, which may need more watering for the first year to help them to get established. Plant trees in autumn, if possible, so they can benefit from natural rainwater as their roots reach down into the soil.

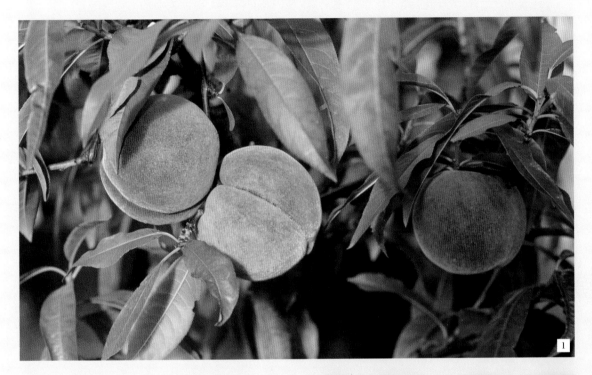

- **Juicy fruits are best** The phytochemical content, especially the carotenoids, of peaches is highest in fruits that are really ripe when harvested. Supermarket peaches are often picked earlier when firm and less likely to be damaged in transit, greatly reducing their nutritional quality. Stored in cool conditions, they are also susceptible to 'chilling injury', which gives peaches an unpleasant, mealy texture. Mealy fruits are less healthy, too, because they have lower levels of phytochemicals, as well as tasting dreadful.

- **Eat the skin** There are two to three times more phytochemicals in the skin than in the flesh of a peach. Beta-carotene levels are up to five times higher, so keep the skin on for optimal nutrition.

- **Store the fruits** Polyphenol levels in peaches rise during storage. Carotenoids increase significantly in the first few days, while polyphenols remain largely unchanged. The carotenoids then stay at a more or less constant level for about two weeks during storage. However, canned peaches lose 30–45 per cent of their polyphenols during processing.

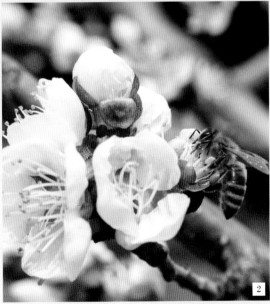

1. *Juicy, ripe peaches have more carotenoids than fruits harvested earlier, when they are firm.* 2. *During a cool early season, if you see that few pollinators, such as bees, are visiting the flowers, you will need to pollinate them by hand.*

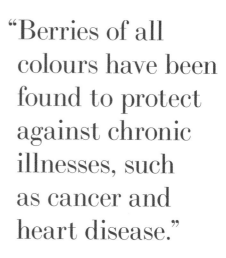

"Berries of all colours have been found to protect against chronic illnesses, such as cancer and heart disease."

1

Berries

Expensive to buy in the shops, most berries are easy to grow and will supply you with a range of health benefits in return for your efforts. Where space is tight, grow plants in containers or a raised bed on a patio or terrace, and include as wide a range as possible.

Strawberries, blackberries, blueberries, blackcurrants, redcurrants, bilberries, loganberries, gooseberries, Chilean guavas, jostaberries, grapes. Just as berries come in different shapes and sizes, so the variety of phytochemicals they contain offer a range of benefits, which you can enjoy by growing as many types as you have space for.

Berries have high levels of antioxidant activity, and a multitude of studies show how they can help prevent chronic health problems, such as cardiovascular diseases, cancer, inflammation, diabetes and age-related diseases. Berries are expensive to buy in the shops but most are easy to grow, supplying you with phytochemicals throughout summer and autumn.

One of the key phytochemicals in berries, such as blackberries, strawberries and raspberries, are ellagitannins, which have anti-inflammatory properties and help to protect against cancer. Blueberries and lingonberries are great sources of resveratrol, a particularly potent antioxidant, most famous for its health-boosting properties in red wine, while dark purple and red fruits contain anthocyanins (see pages 20–21), especially in their skins. Other important phytochemicals found in many berries are quercetin and kaempferol, which protect us against cancer and inflammation of the gut. These are found in especially high quantities in bilberries, cranberries and chokeberries. Any berry you grow will have health benefits, but your cultivation methods can enhance their nutritional value even further.

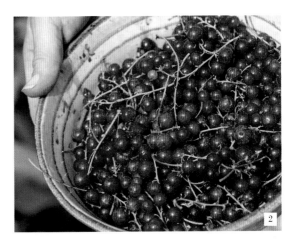

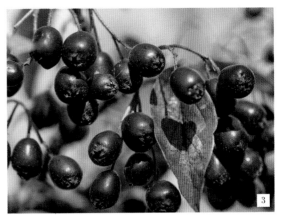

1. *Grow a wide range of berries to benefit from their different phytochemicals.* 2. *Juicy redcurrants are a great source of vitamin C.* 3. *Chokeberries came out top of the berries in a study of the polyphenol content of different types of food.*

HOW TO GROW BERRIES

• **Strawberries** Plant strawberries as bare-root or container-grown plants between autumn and spring. Choose a sunny site and space plants about 30–40cm/12–16in apart. Ensure the base of each crown (where the roots meet the stems) is level with the soil surface when planting. Place straw under the fruit to help prevent the spread of fungal diseases, such as grey mould, which cause the fruits to rot. The fruit may need netting to protect it from birds. In subsequent years the strawberry plants will send out long stems with baby plants at the end, known as 'runners', which can be grown on later in the year to make new plants, or removed, as required. When choosing varieties, consider planting some wild alpine strawberries as they have higher levels of polyphenols.

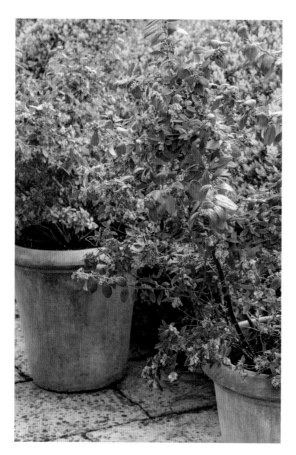

• **Raspberries** Plant raspberries in a sunny site when they are dormant, between late autumn and early spring, either as bare-root or container-grown plants. Plant canes 50–60cm/20–24in apart, and prune new canes to a height of 25cm/10in above ground level. You can grow summer- or autumn-fruiting varieties. For summer-fruiting varieties, prune back canes after they have fruited and tie in the most healthy new shoots to your growing structure (wire and stakes are most commonly used). These canes will fruit the following year. For autumn-fruiting varieties, cut back all the old canes in late winter. Autumn raspberries will fruit on new canes from late summer onwards in the same year. Of the different varieties available, black raspberries have been found to be particularly high in anthocyanins (see pages 20–21).

• **Blackberries** Plant blackberries in a sunny site, spacing plants 2.5–4m/8–13ft apart, and prune existing canes to about 25–30cm/10–12in above soil level. Blackberries can be trained on to wire supports on walls or fences, or up arches, pergolas or trellises. They are vigorous climbers so give them space to grow. Prune old canes to ground level after fruiting and tie in new growth. Grow hybrid blackberries, such as loganberries and tayberries, too, if you have space. All are extremely healthy, but wild varieties have the highest polyphenol levels, although they tend to be less compact and more thorny than their cultivated counterparts.

• **Blackcurrants and jostaberries** Plant blackcurrant and jostaberry bushes in a sunny site as bare-root or container-grown plants between late autumn and early spring, at a distance of approximately 1.5m/5ft apart. After planting, prune back all the stems to about two buds above the soil surface. In future years, cut out any old wood during the winter to strong new shoots, or to the base, to encourage new growth and good cropping.

Blueberries prefer acidic conditions to thrive and fruit well, so grow them in containers in ericaceous compost, unless you have acidic soil (low pH) in your garden.

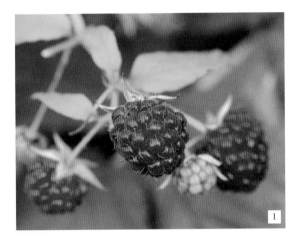

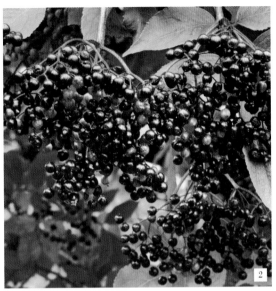

1. *Raspberries are easy to grow in the garden and will reward you with higher phytochemical levels when planted in full sun.*
2. *Elderberries have an exceptionally high polyphenol content, according to a recent research study.*

- **Gooseberries, white- and redcurrants** Grow these fruits as bushes, cordons, or half standards. Plant bare-root or container-grown plants between late autumn and early spring, spacing them about 1.5m/5ft apart. Prune in winter: remove a quarter of the length of the branches on bushes, cutting to an outward-facing bud, and then prune back side-shoots to one to three buds. (Cordons and standards need slightly different pruning methods.)

- **Blueberries** These berries grow best in acidic soil, so if yours is alkaline or neutral grow them in containers using ericaceous compost. Plant bushes 1.5m/5ft apart in the ground and prune lightly. Remove diseased, damaged and older wood to encourage new growth and prolific fruiting. To irrigate the blueberries, collect rainwater, which is likely to be more acidic than tap water. For the highest polyphenol levels select lowbush varieties, or hybrids between highbush and lowbush types, which will be genetically closer to wild blueberries.

- **Elderberries** Containing the second highest levels of polyphenols of any berry, elderberries can be foraged in hedgerows but they are also very easy to grow in the garden. Plants are usually purchased in containers and can be planted at any time of the year, although autumn is probably best. They will become large plants, so give them plenty of space to grow. Prune elderberry bushes hard during the winter to encourage new growth and keep the plants compact. Cut back a third of the growth each year in winter to ground level.

- **Chokeberries (*Aronia*)** Extremely high in polyphenols and pectin (see Health benefits on page 105), chokeberries are very easy to grow in the garden. These hardy plants will reach up to 1.5–2.5m/5–8ft in height and spread, so give them plenty of space. They also have a tendency to sucker, so ensure these shoots are removed, unless you are happy for the plant to spread.

- **Chilean guavas (*Ugni molinae*)** One of my favourite berries, the fruit of Chilean guavas is absolutely delicious and slightly reminiscent of a strawberry. The shrubs are very easy to grow but they prefer a sunny site and slightly acidic conditions, so plant them in containers using ericaceous compost if your soil is alkaline – test it with a pH kit to find out. Plants will eventually grow to a height and spread of approximately 1m/3ft.

GROWING FOR GUT HEALTH

- **Grow wild** Lots of scientific evidence supports the fact that wild berries have higher levels of polyphenols and antioxidant activity than cultivated types. This is partly due to genetic differences and partly because phytochemicals in wild plants are higher because they protect them from the more stressful growing environments they experience. For example, an Italian study showed the total polyphenol level was twice as high and the anthocyanin levels three times higher in wild blueberries compared to cultivated ones. Wild strawberries and blackberries contain three to five times as many polyphenols as the cultivated types. If possible, choose naturally occurring wild varieties and try to mimic their natural growing conditions.

- **Pick berries through the season** The anthocyanin levels of dark red and purple berries increases as the fruits mature, but the total overall polyphenol content and antioxidant level of many berries actually declines during the transition from green to fully ripe stage. Try picking some berries when mid-ripe and others that are fully ripe to gain a range of different types of beneficial phytochemicals.

- **Little treats** Small berries are more nutritious than larger fruits because the skins contain the highest levels of phytochemicals – 100g/3.5oz of small blueberries have a much larger surface area than the same weight of large blueberries, giving them a higher polyphenol rating. Berries from the supermarket are usually large, but they often taste blander, probably due to fewer phytochemicals.

- **Light works** The role of anthocyanins in a plant is to protect it from the sun's rays. Consequently, plants grown under stronger sunlight have higher levels, so site yours in full sun, rather than part-shade, for the richest source of anthocyanins.

- **Cold facts** Studies indicate that the levels of polyphenols in berries are greater when the plants are grown at lower temperatures. Good news if you are in cold northerly regions, or at higher altitudes,

Health benefits

A recent research study's list of the top 100 foods for polyphenol content found some berries had exceedingly high quantities. Chokeberries, native American fruits, and elderberries, which grow in the wild all over Europe in hedgerows and woodland edges, came out top, but other berries were not far behind in the phytochemical stakes.

TOP TEN BERRIES FOR TOTAL POLYPHENOL CONTENT

FRUIT	TOTAL POLYPHENOL CONTENT IN A 100G/ 3.5OZ SAMPLE
Chokeberry	1,756mg/0.062oz
Elderberry	1,359mg/0.048oz
Lowbush blueberry	836mg/0.029oz)
Blackcurrant	758mg/0.027oz
Highbush blueberry	560mg/0.02oz
Blackberry	260mg/0.009oz
Strawberry	235mg/0.008oz
Raspberry	215mg/0.007oz
Black grape	169mg/0.006oz
Green grape	15MG/0.0005OZ

Many nutritious berries are not listed here, but most with dark or brightly coloured fruit will have the highest polyphenol levels.

such as the Scottish raspberries growers and Norwegian cranberry cultivators.

- **Poor soils are best** Phytochemicals are increased in plants grown in nutrient-poor soils, so do not use fertilizers, especially nitrogen or phosphorus. Organic techniques, such as adding manure to the soil, also result in berries with more polyphenols than those given mineral fertilizers. This may be because the plant microbiota (see page 26–27) is enhanced, and the uptake of nutrients is slower.

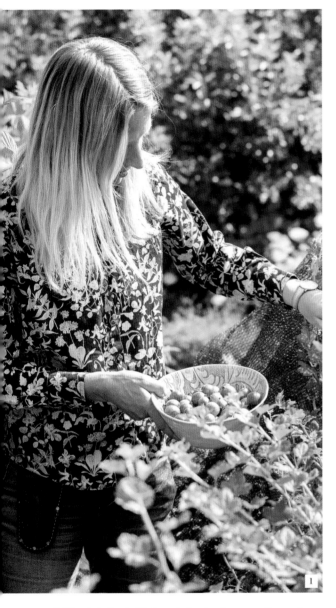

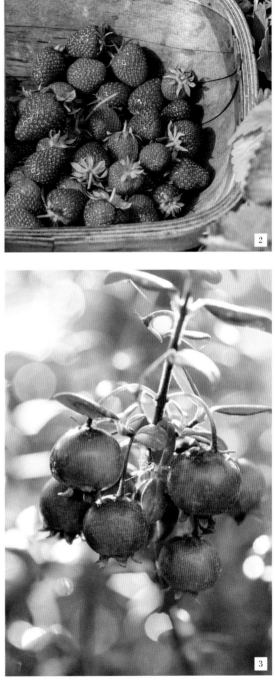

1. *The phytochemical balance in berries changes as they mature, so harvest the fruit throughout the growing season for the greatest diversity.* **2.** *Plant your berries in full sun and exposed locations to increase their phytochemical content.* **3.** *Grow unusual berries, such as these Chilean guavas, to increase diversity in your diet.*

Plums

(Prunus domestica)

Plums and their dried counterparts, prunes, are renowned for their high fibre content, but growing your own trees allows you to source local varieties with higher nutritional value and to harvest the fruits when their phytochemical content is at its peak.

GROWING FOR GUT HEALTH

- **Colour is key** Purple and red plums are much higher in polyphenols than green or yellow varieties, and while the latter are rich in carotenoids, so are the reds and purples – it's just masked by the dark hues of their anthocyanins (see pages 20–21).

- **Go for local varieties** Some research shows local varieties of plum are best when it comes to their nutritional properties. A study into local varieties of the European plum in the Carpathian Mountains found that they had higher levels of antioxidants, minerals and pectin (see Health benefits, page 105).

- **Planting tips** Plant bare-root or container-grown trees in late autumn. Ensure they are at the same depth as they were in their pot or the nursery – you will see the darker soil mark on the stem – and ensure the rootstock union (bump on stem) is above the soil level. If you are planting on an exposed site, your tree may also need staking.

- **Choose a rootstock** St Julien A rootstock is used for most plum trees and produces a tree 3.5–4.5m/12–15ft in height and spread. A more dwarfing rootstock called Pixy is available for small gardens, which produces a 2.5–3m/8–10ft tree.

- **Pollination partners** Many plum trees are self-fertile and do not need a pollination partner to set fruit. Those that do need a pollination partner can often be cross-pollinated by greengages, damsons, or mirabelles, so look around your local area, if needed, to see if there are other trees likely to flower at a similar time.

- **Let the sun in** The anthocyanin content increases when plums are exposed to sunlight, so plant your trees in a sunny spot, and avoid using dark netting, which will shade the fruit, although it may be necessary to protect your crop from birds and

Health benefits

There are about 40 species of plum worldwide but only two are grown commercially: *Prunus domestica* (the European plum), and *Prunus salicina* (the Japanese plum). Both have similar nutritional profiles and are great sources of polyphenols, carotenoids and vitamin C. They also have a high antioxidant activity – higher than peaches or nectarines. Due to their nutritional value, there's been an increasing interest in plums, as they have been found to help increase bone health, improve memory and cognitive skills, and offer anti-inflammatory effects. Some studies also suggest that dried plums may help to protect against osteoporosis.

squirrels. Lay a reflective mulch, such as pale stones or gravel, under the trees to increase the sunlight reaching the fruits on the lower canopy.

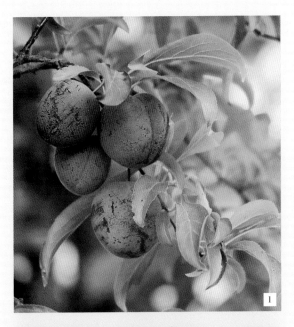

- **Prune wisely** Do not prune plums during the dormant period (late autumn to early spring) as this may expose them to silver leaf and bacterial canker infections at this time of year. Prune instead from late spring to early summer. Plums can be trained as cordons, espaliers or fans against a wall or fence, which will help to expose the fruits to more sunlight.

- **Eat when ripe** The polyphenols and carotenoids in plums increases as the fruit matures, so wait until they are fully ripe before harvesting – their colour and softness are good indicators of this. A study of Japanese plums found the total phenolic content increased by nearly five times, and the carotenoid content by over six times, as they ripened.

- **Keep skins on** With three to nine times the concentration of polyphenols than the flesh, do not remove the skin of your plums before eating.

- **The rise of the prune** Dried plums, or prunes, are good sources of dietary fibre, but the fruits' polyphenol content is greatly reduced as they dry, while the antioxidant level increases. Given that polyphenol content and antioxidant activity are normally closely linked, how is this possible? When some fruits like plums are dried, compounds called melanoidins are formed, which prevent the fruit from rotting while also increasing the antioxidant activity.

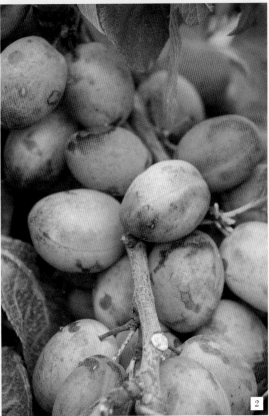

- **Super plums** The Australians have bred a super plum called 'Queen Garnet' with nearly black skin and dark red fruit. It has over twice the anthocyanins of standard plums, and as much as blueberries. We can't buy this variety to grow at home as yet, but for plums with similar nutritional benefits select trees with the darkest fruits you can find.

1. Dark purple plums have the highest polyphenol content.
2. Pick your fruit when it is soft and really ripe for the highest carotenoid and polyphenol values.

Figs

(Ficus carica)

These Mediterranean fruit trees are surprisingly hardy and, given a sunny sheltered spot, they will produce a good crop. Choosing healthier varieties rich in phytochemicals and enjoying the fresh fruits when ripe also offer many more benefits than eating dried shop-bought types.

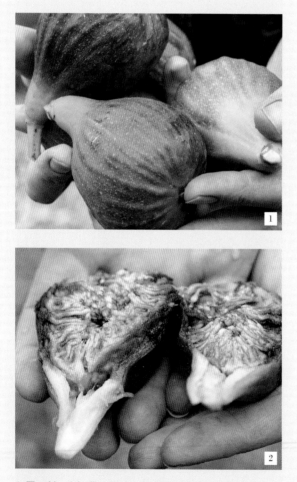

1. The skin of the fig contains the highest concentrations of phytochemicals. 2. There's nothing more delicious than the succulence of a freshly picked fig.

GROWING FOR GUT HEALTH

- **Plump for purple** You can choose figs with purple, yellow or even green flesh, but the dark purple or black varieties are best for our health, with up to three times the phytochemicals of green or yellow varieties. This is largely due to the high anthocyanin content concentrated in the peel. However, green varieties do contain some tannins (like green tea), which are potent antioxidants.

- **Plant by a warm wall** Figs grow well in containers or in a sheltered, sunny spot in the garden. Try training them in a fan shape against a wall to allow as much light as possible to reach the fruits. Plant trees in autumn or spring and make sure they are at the same level as they were planted in the nursery (look for the soil mark on the stem). Fig trees can be very vigorous and thrive in free-draining soil, but they fruit better when their root growth is restricted in a pot or by inserting paving stones or slate on edge around the root ball. Figs grown in a warm Mediterranean climate will crop twice in summer, but outdoor trees grown in cool temperate regions usually only crop once. Remove large unripe fruits at the end of the summer, as they are unlikely to reach maturity, but leave small embryonic fruits, which may ripen the following year.

- **Amazing pollination** The fruit of a fig is a botanical masterpiece. It is actually a mass of hundreds of tiny flowers that are enclosed, inwardly, in a case called

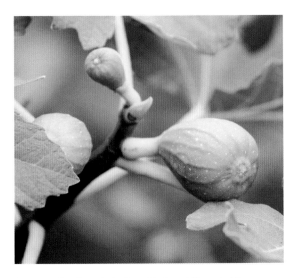

Leave small embryonic fruits on the tree at the end of the year because they may go on to ripen the following season.

the total content is nearly three times higher in the skin than the flesh and, in fresh fruits picked straight from the tree, it is soft and delicious.

- **Ripe benefits** As the fruit ripens, it darkens in colour, softens, and the aroma and sweetness of the fig intensifies. The level of polyphenols and the antioxidant activity also goes up at this stage – fully ripe fruits have twice the polyphenols and two or three times more flavonoids.

- **All dried up** Fresh figs are expensive to buy in the shops and difficult to store, which explains why most are sold in their dried form, but a number of studies has shown dried fruits have a much lower level of polyphenols. This provides yet another good reason to grow your own figs at home, eat them fresh, and save some money too.

a syconium. Figs are fertilized by very small wasps that crawl inside the base of the fig and deposit their eggs there. When the eggs hatch, the young wasps pick up pollen from the flowers, then chew their way out and transfer to another syconium where they fertilize the flowers, and again deposit eggs so the cycle can continue. There are actually over 750 species of fig tree worldwide, each of which has a synergistic relationship with a specific type of wasp. Nature is incredible. However, most figs in cultivation produce fruits that are parthenocarpic – these are seedless and develop without the need for a pollinating wasp.

- **Light, water, temperature** Researchers have observed the phytochemical content of the fruits seems to be higher in drier and hotter conditions, probably due to the stress on the plant which stimulates an increase in defensive phytochemicals. When growing figs, ensure they are in a sunny, sheltered spot to maximize the benefits.

- **Eat the skin** If you've read about other fruit and vegetables in this book, you won't be surprised to read that the skins of figs contain significantly higher levels of polyphenols than the pulp. In fact,

Health benefits

Figs are one of the richest sources of vitamins A, C, and K, as well as potassium and magnesium. They have fantastically high levels of polyphenols and, as a consequence, antioxidant activity. There are 18 different types of polyphenol in figs, including anthocyanins (see pages 20–21), chlorogenic acid (see page 109) and rutin. The latter helps to strengthen blood vessels and improves blood circulation. Figs are also an excellent source of fibre, providing even more than prunes. They contain pectin, a prebiotic fibre that fuels our gut microbes, helping to increase the diversity of beneficial bacteria and promoting good digestive health.

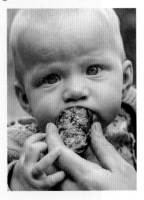

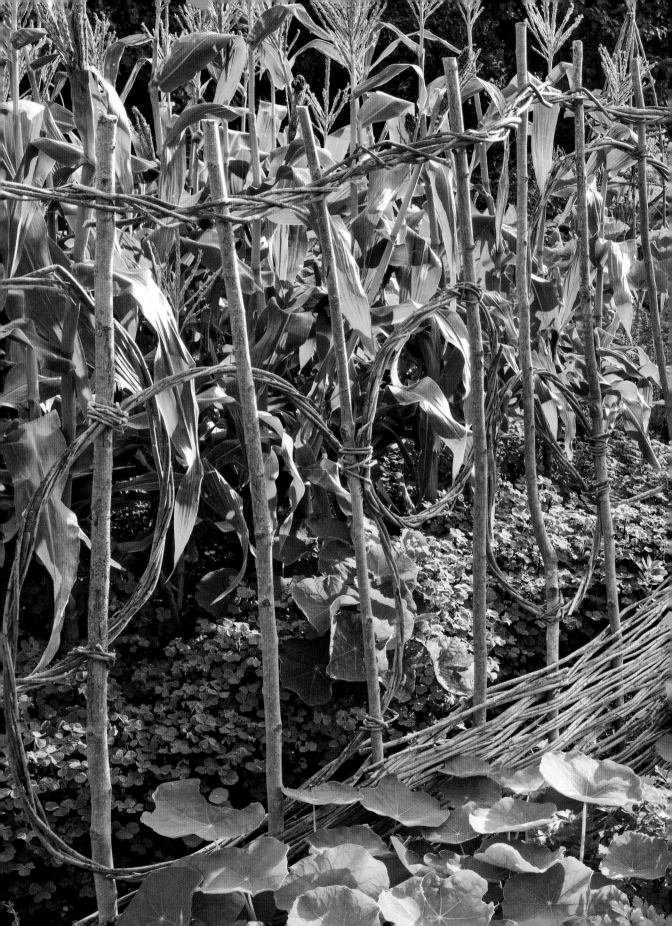

CHAPTER THREE

Grow-for-health Projects

"Now you have learned why home-grown crops can be so good for you, here are some easy projects to get you going."

"Planting one crop, harvesting it, and then planting another maximizes the yield throughout the year from this small bed."

PROJECT 1

Square-metre plot

This project is ideal for a small garden, patio or terrace, and involves planting a diverse range of different health-enhancing crops in a raised bed.

By planting a wide range of crops in just one square metre/yard, you can grow up to 20 different crops over the growing season, planting and harvesting each crop one after the other in succession.

First, you will need to build or buy a 1m x 1m/3ft x 3ft timber-framed raised bed (see page 126 for instructions). The raised bed I have created is 10cm/4in deep. You could make yours a little deeper if you plan to set it on a patio or hard ground where there is no extra soil beneath it. You then divide up the bed into smaller squares of approximately 33cm x 33cm/1ft x 1ft, and use each square to grow a different crop.

The raised bed is an easy-to-organize system and ideal for growing crops successionally. By this I mean planting one crop, then harvesting it when mature and adding a second crop in the same place to harvest a few weeks or months later. This method is most effective for high-yielding plants, such as cut-and-come-again salad leaves, and quick-growing crops, such as radishes, lettuces and spring onions.

By cramming in a diversity of crops, you can make the most of even the tiniest courtyard garden – if it has sufficient sunlight. Planting densely also means the leaves of the crops will shade the soil surface, thereby reducing weed growth and soil-moisture evaporation, so you won't need to water as frequently.

As with all gardening projects for optimum nutrition, try to integrate a range of colour groups into the design, and include some crops with prebiotic fibre to nourish your microbes (see pages 16–19). I have given some suggestions overleaf for you to try.

GROWING TIP

Harvest the foliage of the leafy crops in your plot regularly to ensure the surrounding plants have plenty of space to grow. Removing excess leaves also gives pests, such as slugs and snails, fewer places to hide.

YOU WILL NEED

2 x lengths of timber
(approx. 100 x 200 x
1,200mm/4 x 8 x 48in)

2 x lengths of timber
(approx. 100 x 200 x
1,000mm/4 x 8 x 40in)

4 x galvanized metal brackets

Stainless steel screws

Home-made compost
or topsoil

String and pins

GUIDELINES FOR
PLANTS PER SQUARE

1 plant per square:
cauliflower, cabbages,
aubergines, tomatoes,
kale, sage, rosemary
2 plants per square:
dwarf French beans,
chard, thyme, oregano
4 plants per square:
kohlrabi, Florence fennel,
parsley, dill, shallots,
garlic, lettuces, leeks
9 plants per square:
beetroot, spinach, parsnip,
peas, baby leeks, onions
16 plants per square:
carrots, radishes,
spring onions

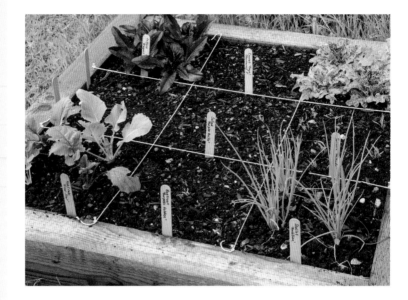

MAKING THE RAISED BED

1. When choosing timber, be cautious about buying treated wood, which may contain toxic chemicals, such as creosote. Some timber suppliers will cut your wood to size on request. We've used softwood railway sleepers, which are durable and relatively cost effective. You will need two lengths of 1,200mm/48in, and two of 1,000mm/40in. Or you could use bricks or stone for a more durable feature.

2. Install your bed in a sunny area and, if necessary, level the ground so the wood lies flat on the surface. Join the sections of timber to form a square and screw in galvanized metal brackets to keep them stable.

3. Add your growing media – we use our own home-made compost, which is ideal, or try a loamy topsoil enriched with organic matter, such as well-rotted manure or mushroom compost. Break down any large lumps from the top layer to create a fine, crumbly surface to sow into.

4. Divide your plot into nine sections using string and pins. Each section designates a square for a different crop – see options left and opposite, and follow the growing advice in the Vegetables & Fruit in Focus chapter (see pages 38–121).

Crops for the bed

Here are suggestions for crop types and the numbers of each to include per square. You will notice that you plant slightly closer than I recommend for planting in the ground, but this is a workable compromise for a raised bed.

EARLY-SEASON CROPS
This group of plants are the first to be sown in early spring. They will be ready to harvest from early to midsummer, when you can replace them with the crops below.

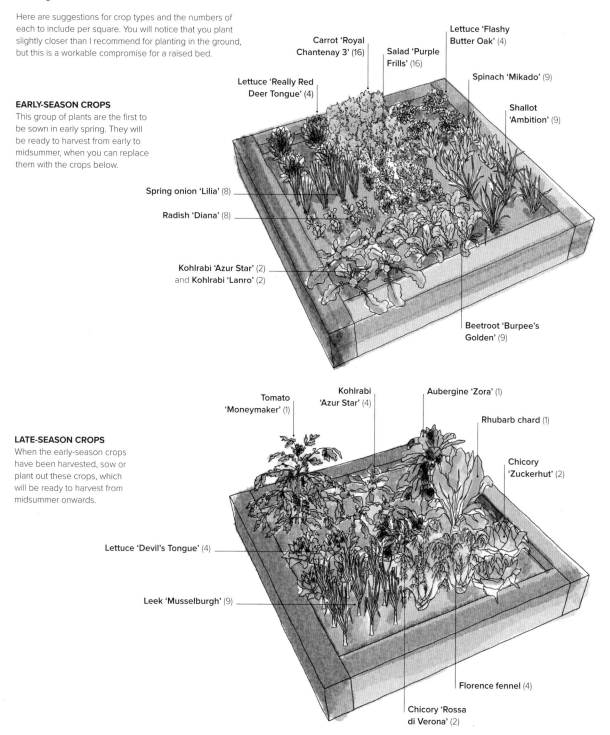

Carrot 'Royal Chantenay 3' (16)

Salad 'Purple Frills' (16)

Lettuce 'Flashy Butter Oak' (4)

Spinach 'Mikado' (9)

Shallot 'Ambition' (9)

Lettuce 'Really Red Deer Tongue' (4)

Spring onion 'Lilia' (8)

Radish 'Diana' (8)

Kohlrabi 'Azur Star' (2) and Kohlrabi 'Lanro' (2)

Beetroot 'Burpee's Golden' (9)

LATE-SEASON CROPS
When the early-season crops have been harvested, sow or plant out these crops, which will be ready to harvest from midsummer onwards.

Tomato 'Moneymaker' (1)

Kohlrabi 'Azur Star' (4)

Aubergine 'Zora' (1)

Rhubarb chard (1)

Chicory 'Zuckerhut' (2)

Lettuce 'Devil's Tongue' (4)

Leek 'Musselburgh' (9)

Florence fennel (4)

Chicory 'Rossa di Verona' (2)

PROJECT 2

Forager's border

This bountiful border packed with different crops allows you to harvest little and often to increase the diversity in your diet and boost gut health.

This project shows how to grow small quantities of a wide range of edibles in a border, so you can forage for produce to make healthy, multi-ingredient meals. It's an excellent way to boost the plant-based variety in our diets to feed our gut microbes and encourage their diversity. I have focused on plants high in polyphenols (see pages 20–21), the phytochemicals that are so beneficial to our microbiota, and included some unusual edibles too. The border I've used is in the protected walled garden, but it would work equally well in a sheltered, sunny space in a garden, or on an allotment. A space close to a wall or a fence is ideal, as it can be used to train wall fruit and edible climbers.

MAKING THE BORDER

1. Divide your border into strips, roughly 50cm/20in wide and 50–100cm/20–39in long. The size of each section is flexible – adapt it to the size and quantity of the crop you choose to grow.

2. Sow or plant each section with a different crop. Cut-and-come-again salads, herbs, and fast-growing crops for successional sowings work well for foraging in small quantities.

3. Use the area by a wall or fence to train fruit trees into fans, espaliers or cordons by tying young, flexible branches to sturdy horizontal wires or a trellis framework.

4. Be creative with your design, treating it like a herbaceous border, with a mix of crop textures, colours and heights. Focus on colourful vegetables, berries and herbs that are high in polyphenols. See overleaf for suggestions of what to grow.

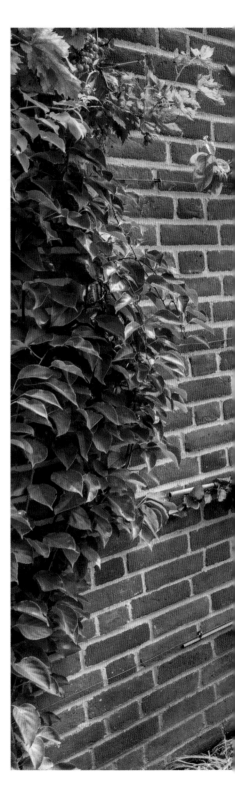

"Make the most of the vertical space in your garden with cordon or espaliered fruit trees and climbing crops."

Planting plan

This illustration shows some examples of the crops you could grow in your Forager's Border, but there are many more that would work equally well. See also the Vegetables & Fruit in Focus chapter (pages 38–121) for other ideas. Check your light levels to ensure the conditions are right for your chosen crops, and make the border bigger or smaller to suit your space.

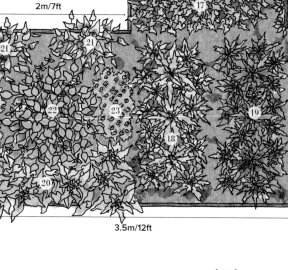

1.5m/5ft

8.5m/28ft

2m/7ft

1.8m/6ft

3.5m/12ft

N

Climbers

1 KIWI (*Actinidia deliciosa*)
How to grow These vigorous climbers need a sunny, sheltered spot to fruit well. Either plant one self-fertile variety or two plants (one male and one female) to ensure pollination occurs.
Health benefits Kiwis are high in a range of polyphenols, including quercetin (see pages 20–21).

2 BLACK GRAPE (*Vitis vinifera*)
How to grow Vigorous climbers, grapes need plenty of space and full sun, plus a sturdy frame for the stems to entwine. Prune in early winter before the sap starts rising.
Health benefits Grapes are high in a polyphenol called resveratrol, a type of anthocyanin (see pages 20–21).

3 PEAR 'BETH' (*Pyrus communis* 'Beth')
How to grow See page 108 for advice.
Health benefits Most of the fibre in pears is pectin, an excellent source of prebiotic fibre, which feeds beneficial gut bacteria.

4 MALABAR SPINACH (*Basella alba*)
How to grow Sow seed indoors in mid- or late spring. Plant out after all risk of frosts has passed. This climbing plant will need wires or a trellis support on a wall or fence. It grows up to 3m/10ft.
Health benefits This is a different species to normal spinach and contains a greater diversity of phytochemicals.

Fruiting shrubs

5 BLACK CHOKEBERRY (*Aronia melanocarpa*)
How to grow Ideally grow in full sun and give plenty of space, as plants reach up to 1.5–2m/5–6ft in height.
Health benefits One of the most abundant sources of polyphenols available, especially high in anthocyanins (see pages 20–21).

6 ELDERBERRY (*Sambucus nigra* f. *porphyrophylla* 'Eva')
How to grow An easy-to-grow shrub, it reaches up to 2–3m/6ft 6in–10ft and will ultimately need plenty of space.
Health benefits The berries are ranked one of the most abundant sources of polyphenols available. The edible flowers are also very high in phytochemicals (see pages 16–21).

Perennial herbs

7 PURPLE SAGE
(*Salvia officinalis* 'Purpurascens')
How to grow Grow this evergreen sub-shrub in full sun and well-drained soil. Plants are fairly drought tolerant.
Health benefits An excellent source of polyphenols, including rosmarinic acid, which gut microbes help to break down.

8 ROSEMARY (*Salvia rosmarinus*)
How to grow Grow in full sun and well-drained soil. This mid-sized shrub grows up to 1.5m/5ft in height.
Health benefits High in polyphenols, such as caffeic acid and rosmarinic acid, which have antioxidant and anti-inflammatory properties.

9 THYME (*Thymus vulgaris*)
How to grow Grow in full sun and well-drained soil. Space plants about 40cm/16in apart, and cut stems regularly to keep these sub-shrubs compact.
Health benefits High in flavonoids and polyphenols, especially rosmarinic acid (see Rosemary, above).

Annuals

10 NASTURTIUM (*Tropaeolum*)
How to grow Choose climbing or bush varieties and sow seed in the border in mid-spring. Provides an abundance of edible flowers. Can be susceptible to aphids.
Health benefits Edible flowers are high in carotenoids and polyphenols, which have antioxidant and anti-inflammatory properties. The edible leaves are also rich in vitamin C.

11 SCULPIT (*Silene vulgaris*)
How to grow An easy-to-grow perennial, sow seed in modules indoors in mid-spring and plant out in late spring or early summer after the frosts.
Health benefits The leaves have significant antioxidant activity and polyphenol content.

12 BUCK'S HORN PLANTAIN
(*Plantago coronopus*)
How to grow Sow seed in the border in mid-spring once the soil has warmed up. Use as a cut-and-come-again salad vegetable, harvesting the leaves as needed.
Health benefits Research shows it is a good source of unusual types of caffeic acid (see also Rosemary, above).

13 SPRING ONION 'LILIA'
How to grow Sow seed directly outside at regular intervals from mid-spring onwards, for crops throughout the growing season.
Health benefits With over four times the concentration of phytochemicals of standard white onions, the red varieties also have anthocyanins (see pages 20–21).

14 ITALIAN DANDELION 'RED RIB'
(*Cichorium intybus* 'Red Rib')
How to grow Sow seed inside in modules from early spring and plant out from mid- to late spring.
Health benefits Italian dandelions are a great source of inulin, a type prebiotic fibre (see page 19). The foliage is also high in phytochemicals, such as lutein and quercetin (see pages 20–21).

15 SWEET CICELY (*Myrrhis odorata*)
How to grow Sow seed in spring or autumn indoors and plant out from spring onwards.
Health benefits Sweet cicely, like many herbs, has high levels of polyphenols and antioxidant activity.

16 PERILLA (*Perilla frutescens*)
How to grow Sow seeds from early spring onwards indoors – it needs warmth to germinate successfully. Plant out when the frosts are over.
Health benefits Try the purple form, which is an excellent source of polyphenols, including rosmarinic acid (see Rosemary, left) luteolin, which helps protect against cancer and heart disease, and quercetin (see pages 20–21).

17 CUCAMELON (*Melothria scabra*)
How to grow Sow seed indoors in late spring, and plant out after the frosts.
Health benefits Rich in flavonoids, tannins and saponin, which are good sources of antioxidants and help regulate our microbes.

18 MEXICAN TREE SPINACH
(*Chenopodium giganteum*)
How to grow Sow seed indoors in mid-spring in a light, warm environment. Plant out after the risk of frosts has passed. This plant self-seeds freely so you will probably only need to buy and sow the seed once!
Health benefits Mexican tree spinach has a startling pink bloom to the leaves – the brightly coloured pigments are an indicator of its high polyphenol content.

19 AZTEC BROCCOLI
(*Chenopodium nuttalliae*)
How to grow Sow seed indoors mid-spring and plant out after the frosts.
Health benefits Aztec broccoli is closely related to Mexican tree spinach. It's a good source of polyphenols, such as flavonoids, tannins and saponin.

20 CAPE GOOSEBERRY
(*Physalis peruviana*)
How to grow Sow seed indoors in mid-spring and plant out after the frosts.
Health benefits Fruits contain unusual types of polyphenol, such as withanolides, which have anti-inflammatory and anti-cancer effects, as well as carotenoids (see pages 20–21).

21 TOMATILLO (*Physalis ixocarpa*)
How to grow Sow seed indoors in mid-spring and plant out after the frosts.
Health benefits Tomatillos contain withanolides (see Cape gooseberry, above)

22 RUNNER BEAN 'CZAR'
How to grow Sow seed indoors in mid-spring and plant out after the frosts, or sow directly outside in late spring.
Health benefits Packed full of prebiotic fibre, resistant starch and polyphenols.

23 FRENCH MARIGOLD (*Tagetes patula*)
How to grow Sow seed indoors in a warm, light place from early to mid-spring and plant out after the frosts.
Health benefits The edible flowers contain a polyphenol called laricitin which has anti-inflammatory and antioxidant qualities.

24 CHICORY 'ZUCKERHUT'
AND 'ROSSA DI VERONA'
How to grow Sow seed from early to midsummer indoors and plant out after the red spring onions have been harvested.
Health benefits The leaves are a great source of polyphenols, including quercetin, kaempferol and apigenin. Chicory root also contains prebiotic fibre (see pages 16–19).

25 LETTUCE 'DEVIL'S TONGUE'
How to grow Sow in early summer indoors and plant out after the red onions have been harvested.
Health benefits Contains polyphenols, such as quercetin, rutin and kaempferol. Red lettuces also contain anthocyanins (see pages 20–21).

PROJECT 3

Ten prebiotic fibre superfoods

Selected for their prebiotic fibre content, these delicious crops will feed your gut microbes and keep your digestive and immune systems healthy.

All plants contain fibre but some are a particularly good sources of the type that feeds the beneficial bacteria in our gut. This prebiotic fibre cannot be digested in the small intestine, and instead passes into the gut where it is fermented by our friendly bacteria (see also pages 16–19).

Prebiotics play a critical role in ensuring that we have a diverse and balanced community of bacteria in our gut. They help to keep our digestive systems healthy, soothing any inflammation and enhancing the immune system, which in turn wards off diseases. They also help our bodies to absorb important minerals, such as magnesium and calcium, that support strong bone and tooth development. In addition, studies show prebiotic fibre has many other benefits, reducing the risk of heart disease and cancer, helping to balance hormones, boosting our mood and mental wellbeing, and much more.

The best edible plants to grow for gut health are those with high levels of fructans, which is a form of prebiotic fibre. Plants produce fructans to help them to store energy, which can then be used during periods of stress, such as when temperatures take a dive or soil water levels are low. Usually found in plants' underground storage organs, such as tubers or bulbs, fructans normally come in one of two forms: inulin or fructooligosaccharides (see page 19). Fructans-rich plants include the sunflower family (see pages 60–69), the onion family (see pages 40–47), and grasses, which comprise grains such as wheat and oats.

GROWING TIP

Applying nitrogen-rich fertilizers has a negative effect on fructans levels in plants. To maximize the prebiotic content of these crops, avoid using these types of feed and do not add manure to the soil where the plants will be grown.

Clockwise from top left *Cardoon, garlic, globe artichoke and yacon. All are rich in fibre, providing fuel for your gut microbes and adding diversity to your diet.*

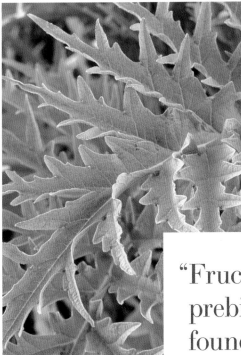

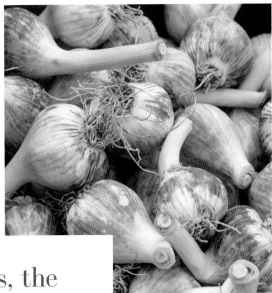

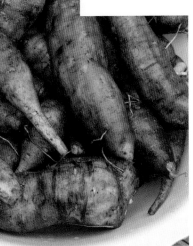

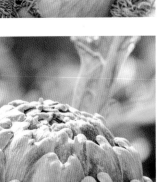

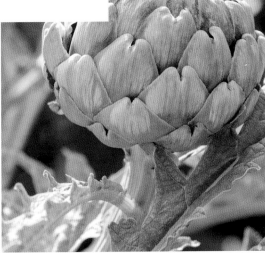

"Fructans, the prebiotic fibre found in plants, helps the body absorb minerals that keep our bones strong."

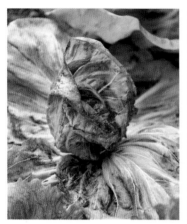

Chicory

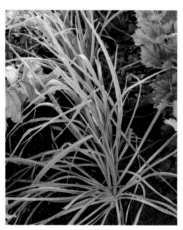

Salsify

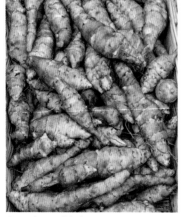

Jerusalem artichoke

Top ten prebiotics

Here are ten easy-to-grow edible plants that are packed with prebiotic fibre for your gut microbes. If you can, grow them all to enrich your diet with as much diversity as possible. Many can be harvested in winter, providing some welcome seasonal bounty.

1. Root chicory

All chicory roots are extremely high in inulin, the most common ingredient found in prebiotic supplements. This plant is very easy to grow at home, and it is best eaten as a wholefood. There are many different types of chicory, but the one to grow for the roots is *Cichorium intybus* var. *sativum*, simply called root chicory in many seed catalogues. Use the roots in soups and stews. It's also traditionally dried and ground to make a coffee substitute.

Growing advice
Sow seed directly outside in late spring or early summer. Plant at a depth of 1–2cm/½–1in and thin the seedlings to 15cm/6in apart when they have a few leaves. Avoid sowing too early as plants have a tendency to bolt when daylight hours increase. Harvest from late autumn to early winter.

2. Salsify

Despite not often appearing on lists of recommended prebiotic vegetables, salsify (*Tragopogon porrifolius*) has a very high fructans content (see pages 20–21). It may be difficult to find in the supermarkets, but that's not a problem for gardeners. Commonly called the 'vegetable oyster', salsify is supposed to be reminiscent of that delicacy, but personally I think it tastes more like coconut. The roots also have a crunchy water-chestnut texture.

Growing advice
Sow seed directly into a prepared bed in mid-spring once the soil has warmed up.

Sow to a depth of 1–2cm/½–1in and thin plants to 10cm/4in apart once they have developed a few leaves. Harvest the roots from autumn onwards and roast or add to stews and casseroles.

3. Jerusalem artichokes

Notoriously known as 'fartychokes', Jerusalem artichokes can produce unwanted gas if eaten in large quantities. When eaten in moderation, however, your gut bacteria are unlikely to complain because they have excellent prebiotic qualities. They are also easy to grow and require very little maintenance once established, but they do have a tendency to spread if you don't harvest all the tubers.

Growing advice
Plant tubers out in mid-spring about 30cm/12in apart and 10-15cm/4–6in deep. For further planting advice, see page 64.

4. Yacon

Yacon (*Smallanthus sonchifolius*), also known as jícama, aricoma, yacon strawberry and *poire de terre* in French, is a tuberous edible from the Andes. A close relative of the sunflower, yacon is an amazing plant, with huge underground tubers that taste really sweet. Each plant produces large quantities of tasty tubers so you will only need two or three plants to feed a family. You can include these vegetables in fruit salads, or just eat them raw as a snack.

Growing advice
Grow yacon from tubers planted in pots indoors in early spring, and plant outside in late spring or early summer after the frosts, spacing them approximately 80cm/32in apart. You can plant a quick-growing crop, such as radishes or spring onions, between them early in the season.

5. Globe artichokes

Globe artichokes have a high fructans and polyphenol content and greater antioxidant activity than almost any other vegetable. These perennials are also no trouble to grow and their architectural flower spikes look fabulous in the garden. Harvest the flower buds before they open and cook them lightly to preserve their nutritional value. Remove each scale and eat the succulent bases – the inner scales are so tender they can often be eaten whole. In the centre of the flower bud is the artichoke heart, the part of the plant with the greatest concentration of phytochemicals.

Growing advice
Globe artichokes can be grown from seed sown in spring, but most people buy young container-grown plants to plant directly in the ground in spring or autumn. (For more growing advice, see pages 62–63).

6. Garlic

Garlic is known for its high fructans content, which is stored in the bulb as an energy reserve when plants are dormant. Although we eat garlic in small quantities. it is relatively rich in this form of fibre when compared to most other vegetables, so a little still has a positive effect. It also includes sulphur compounds and other polyphenols to its credit (see also pages 20–21).

Growing advice
Plant cloves directly outside from autumn until early spring. Plant approximately 15cm/6in apart and 5cm/2in deep and harvest the bulbs from early to midsummer.

7. Chinese artichokes

Chinese artichokes (*Stachys affinis*) are delicious, slightly sweet, knobbly tubers with a texture similar to water chestnuts. They contain high quantities of stachyose, a form of fructans that our gut microbes can ferment. Eat them raw, sautéed or steamed.

Growing advice
Plant seed tubers from late autumn to early spring, approximately 8cm/3¼in deep and 30cm/12in apart. Plants require very little maintenance until they are ready to harvest from late autumn to early winter. They can be a little fiddly to harvest, but produce prolific quantities of tubers.

8. Scorzonera

Also known as black salsify, *Scorzonera hispanica* is very closely related to regular salsify and has a similar delicious flavour. Another member of the sunflower family, it produces long, black taproots that are rich

in inulin (see page 19). In the second year of growth, plants bear starry yellow flowers, which are also edible and look lovely in salads.

Growing advice
Grow as for salsify, sowing seed outside in mid-spring once the soil has warmed up. Harvest the roots from autumn onwards; use in soups and stews, or roast or steam them.

9. Cardoon

I've never seen cardoon (*Cynara cardunculus*) for sale in UK supermarkets, but it is popular in some European countries. It's a close relative of the globe artichoke, but you eat the stems rather than the flower buds. Relatively high in fructans, traditionally the stems are often blanched as they grow, using cardboard or hessian sacking tied around them with string in late summer. This makes the cardoon more succulent, but also probably reduces the phytochemical and fibre content. Harvest by cutting bundles of the stems at the bases and cook lightly. The flavour is quite earthy, similar to its botanical cousin the globe artichoke.

Growing advice
You can sow seed in pots indoors in early spring, but because plants may take a couple of years to get established most people grow them from young plants, which are planted outside in spring or autumn. Mature cardoons are enormous, so leave approximately 1.5m/5ft between plants. Like globe artichokes, they need very little attention subsequently. Harvest the stems in late summer. Cut back the old foliage in winter or early spring and new leaves will soon emerge as the temperatures rise.

10. Oca

A tuberous vegetable from South America. oca (*Oxalis tuberosa*) produces brightly coloured, crunchy tubers that are high in prebiotic fructans. They taste similar to a lemony potato and can be eaten raw, roasted or steamed.

Growing advice
Plant tubers in pots indoors in mid-spring and plant out 60–90cm/2–3ft apart after all risk of frost has passed. Leave the tubers in the ground until after the first frosts in late autumn, and harvest the tubers when all the foliage has died back.

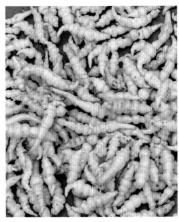
Chinese artichokes

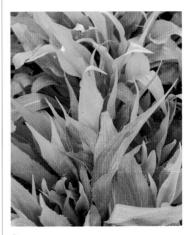
Scorzonera

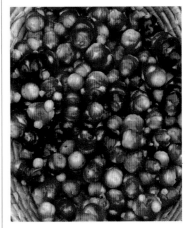
Oca

PROJECT 4

Rainbow pots

This rainbow of tasty, nutrient-rich edibles is easy to grow in large pots on a patio or balcony and provides a succession of delicious crops.

To help you eat a rainbow (see pages 20–21), try these simple edibles in pots. I have used five containers, each representing a different colour group — purple, red, orange and yellow, green, and white — to provide a range of different types of fibre, vitamins, minerals and phytochemicals.

These pretty pots will fit into a small space and I've chosen plants that do well when confined to containers. You can follow my choices (overleaf) or grow whatever you fancy eating, as long as it's suitable for a pot. Most of the plants can be grown from seed sown in spring and then planted into their final containers to grow on. A few take slightly longer to get established and are best bought in spring as young plants if they are to produce crops in the first year. I also recommend planting all your crops simultaneously — that way you can arrange them most effectively in their containers, and they should knit together naturally as they grow.

CHOOSING CROPS FOR POTS

Growing plants in pots is a great opportunity to get creative and choose unusual crop varieties — I've selected a range with different shapes and textures that look beautiful on a patio, as well as being healthy and nutritious. These include agretti — a delicious succulent from coastal parts of the Mediterranean, similar to samphire; Italian dandelion, which is actually a form of chicory and really beneficial for gut health; and perilla, a spicy herb from the mint family.

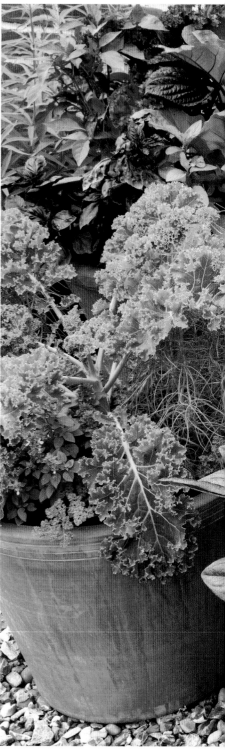

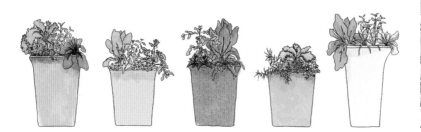

GROWING TIP

Feed all your pots weekly with
a seaweed-based plant feed,
fermented plant fertilizer or compost
tea (see page 151) to boost beneficial
microbes on the plants and in the
growing media, and to increase
the phytochemical content
of your produce.

YOU WILL NEED

5 x large pots

General-purpose peat-free compost

Seed trays, pots and growing modules

Seeds and/or plants of your choice from the different colour groups

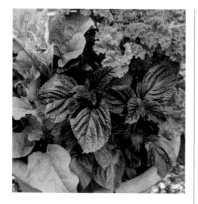

Purple pot

1 x Kale 'Red Curled'
1 x Black peppermint
1 x *Perilla frutescens*
1 x Chilli 'Black Hungarian'
1 x Aubergine 'Zora'
2 x Basil 'Red Rubin'

How to grow

• In early spring, sow the chilli, basil and aubergine seed in modules indoors. Keep seedlings moist and move to larger pots as they grow; keep inside until after the frosts.
• For the kale and perilla, follow the advice above, but start seed off in mid-spring.
• Buy a young peppermint plant in spring; mint is invasive but shouldn't be a problem in a pot for one season.
• After the frosts, plant your edibles outside in a large container in a warm, sunny spot.

Aftercare

• Water as necessary but do not overwater, so that plants are a little stressed.
• Pinch out the stem tips of the perilla to keep it bushy and compact.
• Cover the kale with fine mesh to prevent attacks by cabbage-white butterfly, or use an organically certified biological control such as *Bacillus thuringiensis*.
• Stake the chilli if needed during the growing season and tie in the stems. Pinch out the growing tips when plants are 15–20cm/6–8in high to encourage compact growth and better fruiting.

Harvesting tips

• Pick the perilla and peppermint leaves as needed for multi-ingredient meals.
• Harvest the aubergine's small, dark fruits in late summer and autumn. The chillies will change colour from green to dark purple. Harvest them at different stages for their different types of phytochemical.

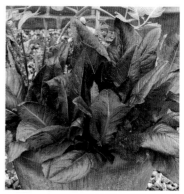

Red pot

1 x Rhubarb chard
1 x Tomato 'Moneymaker'
1 x Dandelion 'Red Rib'
  (*Cichorium intybus* 'Red Rib')
3 x Lettuce 'Devil's Tongue'

How to grow

• In early or mid-spring, sow the tomato and lettuce seed in small pots or modules indoors, and move the plants into larger pots as they grow, but keep them inside.
• Sow the Italian dandelion and chard in mid-spring in pots or modules inside or out (these plants are hardy), transferring them into larger pots as they grow.
• In late spring, or when all risk of frost has passed, plant your crops outside in a large container in a warm, sunny spot. Stake the tomato with a tall cane and tie the main stem to it with soft twine.

Aftercare

• Pinch out any shoots growing between the main and side stems of the tomato regularly, and keep tying in the main stem to its stake as the plant grows.
• The Italian dandelion has a tendency to bolt: remove the flowering inflorescences at the base if they emerge, or keep them and add the edible flowers to salads.

Harvesting tips

• Harvest the chard leaves regularly to add to your dishes; this also prevents them from blocking light to the other plants.
• Pick the Italian dandelion and lettuce leaves when large enough and add them to salads. Harvest the tomatoes when ripe in late summer and early autumn. Wait until the tomatoes are red before harvesting them to maximize the levels of the beneficial phytochemical lycopene (see page 94).

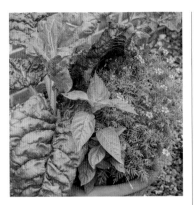

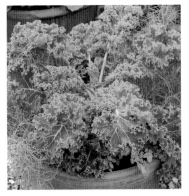

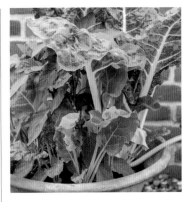

Orange & yellow pot

1 x Tomato 'Datterino Yellow'
2 x Chard 'Pirol'
1 x Chilli 'Lemon Drop'
3 x *Tagetes* 'Lemon Gem'

How to grow

- In early or mid-spring, sow the tomato, chilli and African marigold (*Tagetes*) seed in small pots or modules indoors, and repot as they grow but keep them inside.
- Sow the chard in mid-spring in pots or modules inside or out (these plants are hardy), transferring the seedlings into larger pots as they grow.
- Plant into their final pot after all risk of frost has passed, and set outside in a warm, sunny, sheltered spot. Add a cane to stake the tomato plant.

Aftercare

- Pinch out the shoots growing between the main and side stems of the tomato regularly, and tie the main stem to its stake.
- Pinch out tips of the marigold to encourage compact bushy growth. The flowers are edible and this plant should also act as a companion plant to attract pollinators and deter whitefly.
- Stake the chilli if needed during the growing season. Pinch out the growing tips when plants are 15–20cm/6–8in tall to encourage compact growth and more abundant fruiting.

Harvesting tips

- Pick the chard leaves regularly when about the size of your hand and steam or stir-fry.
- Harvest the tomatoes and chillies when ripe in late summer and early autumn.
- Pick the edible marigold flowers regularly to add to salads or use as a garnish.

Green pot

1 x Curly kale 'Dwarf Green Curled'
2 x Agretti
1 x Parsley 'Champion Moss Curled'
1 x Parsley French

How to grow

- In early spring, sow the agretti seed on the surface of small pots or seed trays and cover very lightly with soil. Keep moist and pot on as the seedlings grow, but keep them indoors.
- In mid-spring, sow the kale and parsleys in pots or modules inside or out (these plants are hardy), and move them into larger pots as they grow.
- When all risk of frost has passed, plant in their final pot outside in a warm, sunny or partly shaded area.

Aftercare

- Cover the kale with fine mesh to prevent attacks by cabbage-white butterfly, or use an organically certified biological control, such as *Bacillus thuringiensis*.
- Keep the pots moist but do not overwater them – the plants will produce more phytochemicals if slightly stressed.

Harvesting tips

- Harvest the kale leaves when mature rather than as baby leaf, as the larger foliage has higher phytochemical levels.
- Pick the tips of the agretti when the leaves are young and succulent – lightly steam them or eat them raw in salads. The plant should continue to produce new growth all summer for harvesting.
- Pick the parsley leaves when they are young. The more you pick, the more the plant will produce, but do not strip plants completely in one picking.

White pot

2 x Swiss chard 'Fordhook Giant'
3 x Beetroot 'Albino'
5 x Shallot 'Ambition'
1 x Pepper 'Amy'

How to grow

- In early spring, sow the shallot and pepper seed indoors in small pots or modules. Sow the shallots in groups of 5–6 seeds in small pots, or alternatively plant shallot sets in autumn. Shallots grow well in groups; no need to thin them, the bulbs will naturally push each other apart as they grow.
- In mid-spring, sow the chard and beetroot in pots or modules inside or out (these plants are hardy), transferring them into larger pots as they grow. The beetroot can be sown individually or in a group of 3–4 seeds, which can then be planted out together in the final container.
- When all risk of frost has passed, plant in their final container outside in a warm, sunny spot.

Aftercare

- Remove dead foliage to increase air circulation around the plants, which reduces the risk of fungal diseases.
- Stake the pepper if needed during the growing season. Pinch out the growing tip when the plant is 15–20cm (6–8in) high to encourage better fruiting.

Harvesting tips

- Harvest the chard leaves regularly to prevent them blocking light.
- Pull the shallots when the foliage starts to wither. Cure the shallots in the sun to maximize their phytochemical content.
- Harvest the beetroots when you see the necks forcing their way out of the soil.
- Harvest the long peppers from midsummer to early autumn.

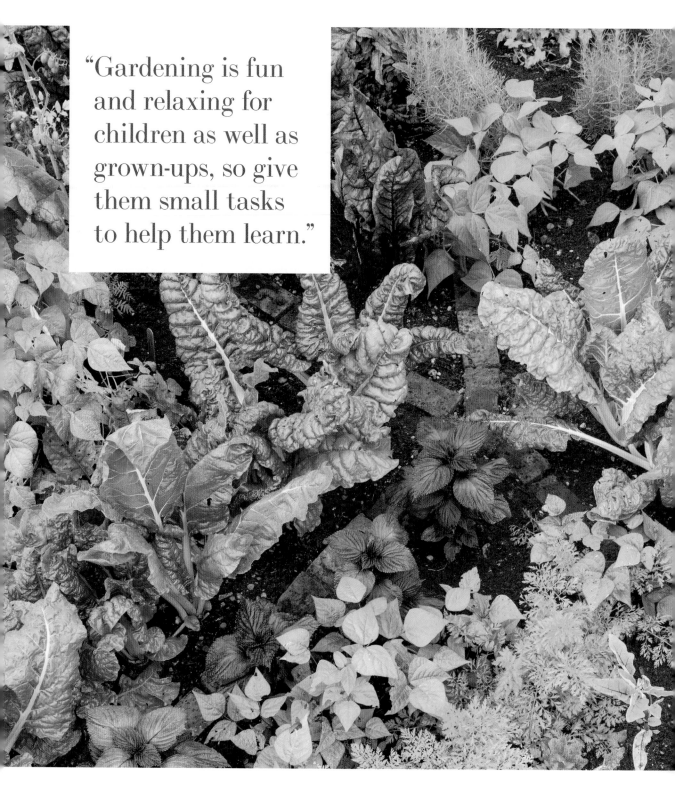

"Gardening is fun and relaxing for children as well as grown-ups, so give them small tasks to help them learn."

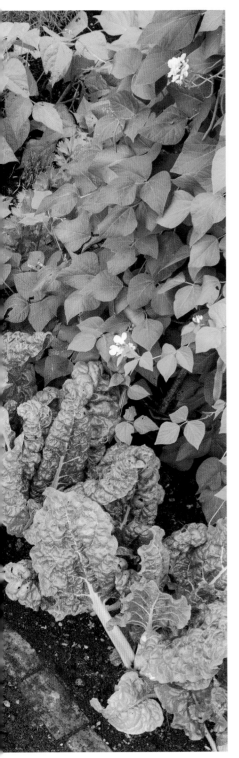

PROJECT 5

Rainbow allotment plot

Divide up an allotment or patch in your garden to grow a range of colourful crops that will increase the diversity of phytochemicals on your menu.

This project demonstrates how to design and grow a plot planted with a rainbow of colourful edibles. The plot is divided into five segments, each containing crops of a different colour that represent different types of health-promoting phytochemicals (see pages 19–21). This is a fun, attractive project that you can put together on your own, or with your friends and family. If you have children, let the little ones choose which coloured plants they would like to grow, and share their enjoyment and surprise in discovering unusual produce. I have suggested some wonderful crops overleaf that my family has enjoyed growing and eating, but feel free to go off-piste and experiment with whatever you fancy.

MAKING A RAINBOW ALLOTMENT PLOT

Our rainbow allotment plot is 5m x 4m/16ft x 13ft, which is an ample space to grow a wide range of different crops. Simply divide your plot up into five sections using aged bricks, stone, timber or other edible plants, such as herbs, for decorative effect.

As with other projects in this book, think about crops you can sow regularly throughout the growing season for a continuous crop (successional sowing). Also include fast-maturing edibles that will fit between slower-growing vegetables; 'follow-on' crops that are planted after the first crops have been harvested to extend the season; and crops that will be available for picking over winter. Flowering companion plants, such as borage, nasturtiums, and marigolds (*Calendula* and *Tagetes*), can also be included to attract pollinators, deter pests, or act as decoys by attracting pests to them rather than to your crops.

Purple/blue

1 PERILLA FRUTESCENS
Sow seed in mid-spring indoors and pot on as seedlings mature. Plant out after the frosts. Keep plants moist. Encourage compact bushy growth by removing the stem tips and harvesting regularly.

2 DWARF FRENCH BEAN 'PURPLE TEEPEE'
Sow seed inside in mid- or late spring in medium-sized pots. Sow two seeds per pot and thin to the strongest seedling. Plant outside after the frosts. Alternatively, sow directly in the ground after the frosts.

3 CARROT 'DEEP PURPLE'
Sow seed directly in the ground from mid-spring onwards once the soil has warmed up. Protect from carrot root fly by covering the crop with fine netting.

4 AUBERGINE 'ZORA'
Sow seed inside in pots or modules in early spring. Pot on and delay planting out until all risk of frost has passed.

5 LETTUCE 'FLASHY BUTTER OAK'
Sow seed in pots or modules inside from early spring. Transplant into modules or small pots when seedlings have a few leaves. Pot on until plants have established a good root ball, after which they can be transferred to the plot.

6 PURPLE FENNEL
Can be sown from seed in spring or autumn, or buy young plants in pots to grow on. Fennel is likely to self-seed freely in subsequent years.

Red

7 RHUBARB CHARD
Sow seed directly outside in the bed in mid-spring. Thin seedlings to approximately 40cm/16in apart. Harvest regularly to ensure the leaves don't block out too much sunlight from the other plants.

8 ONION 'RED BARON'
Plant sets directly in the ground in autumn or spring (see pages 42–43).

9 BEETROOT 'BULL'S BLOOD'
In mid-spring, sow seed inside or outside in pots or modules. Try multi-sowing in groups of 3–4 seeds per module and plant out when seedlings are large enough to handle.

10 SORREL 'RED VEINED'
Sow seed directly in mid-spring. If you sow thinly the seedlings will not need thinning. Harvest as a cut-and-come-again crop.

11 LETTUCE 'DEVIL'S TONGUE'
Follow advice for Lettuce 'Flashy Butter Oak'.

12 OCA
Start oca tubers off in pots in early spring and plant out after the frosts (see page 135).

Orange/yellow

13 TOMATO 'SUNGOLD'
Sow seed in small pots early spring inside. Pot on and plant out after the frosts (see pages 94–5).

14 TAGETES 'GOLDEN GEM'
Sow seed from early to mid-spring inside in small pots or modules. Plant out after the frosts. Remove stem tips to encourage compact bushy growth. The flowers are edible and help to attract pollinators.

15 CLIMBING FRENCH BEAN 'NECKARGOLD'
Grow as for dwarf French bean 'Purple Teepee' (see left).

16 BEETROOT 'BURPEE'S GOLDEN'
Grow as for beetroot 'Bull's Blood' (see left).

17 CHARD 'PIROL'
Grow as for rhubarb chard (see left).

Green

18 DWARF FRENCH BEAN 'TENDERGREEN'
Follow advice for dwarf French bean 'Purple Teepee' (see left).

19 CUCAMELON
Sow 2–3 seeds per pot from mid- to late spring inside. Pot on and plant out after the risk of frost has passed.

20 AGRETTI
Sow indoors in early spring in pots or modules. Pot on as plants grow and plant out after the frosts. Keep plants moist.

21 SPINACH 'MIKADO'
Sow seed directly outside in mid-spring. Sow 2–3 seeds close together and 5–10cm/2–4in apart. Thin to the strongest seedling. Do not sow too late, as it has a tendency to bolt as daylight hours increase. Harvest as a cut-and-come-again vegetable.

22 CHIVES
Sow seed inside in small pots or modules in early spring, and plant out in late spring.

White/brown

23 CELERIAC 'MONARCH'
Sow seed inside in pots or modules in early spring. Seed is very fine, so sow on the surface and do not cover with soil or vermiculite. Transplant seedlings into small pots and plant out after the frosts.

24 RUNNER BEAN 'CZAR'
Sow seed inside from mid- to late spring in medium-sized pots. Sow two seeds per pot and remove the weaker seedling that emerges. Plant out after the frosts.

25 SHALLOT 'AMBITION'
From early to mid-spring, sow seed inside in modules or small pots. Best multi-sown in groups of 5–6 seeds, then pot on as plants grow. Plant out from mid- to late spring.

26 SWISS CHARD 'FORDHOOK GIANT'
Grow as for rhubarb chard (see left).

27 STRAWBERRIES
Plant out bare-root plants from autumn to early spring. Your fruit may need netting to protect it from birds or squirrels.

SUCCESSIONAL CROPS

You can grow these crops before and after those shown on the illustration:
Purple Kale 'Red Curled'; Mangetout 'Shiraz'; Lettuce 'Devil's Tongue'; Mustard greens 'Purple Frills'
Red Radish 'Diana'
Orange/yellow Dwarf French bean 'Berggold'; Green lettuce 'Little Gem'
White Pak choi 'Bonsai'

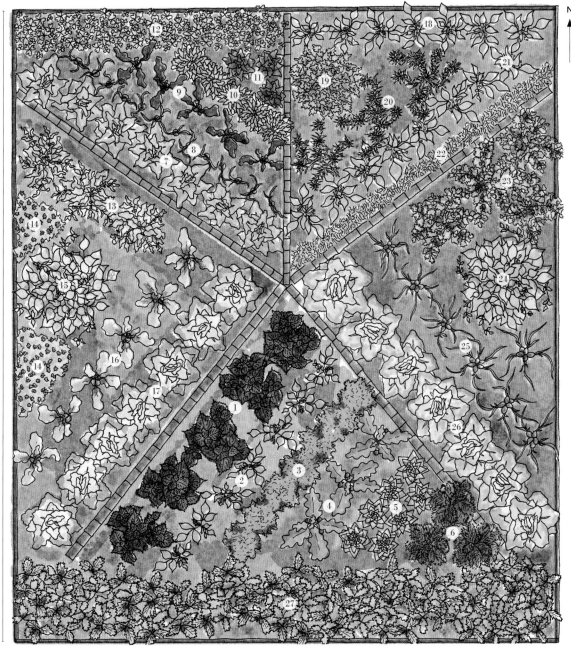

5m/16ft

4m/13ft

Choosing crops for a rainbow allotment

You can be really creative about which crops you grow. I've chosen some of our favourite edibles (see opposite) in our 5m x 4m/16ft x 13ft plot, which feeds my family almost all year, but you can, of course, select other crops from the Vegetables & Fruit in Focus chapter (see pages 38–121).

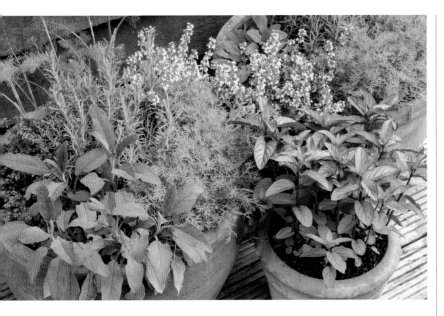

Managing your pots

- **Don't overwater herbs** as most prefer free-draining soil and limiting water will also increase their phytochemical levels — by up to 46 times in the case of basil.

- **Pick herbs regularly** to keep the plants compact and encourage new leaf growth.

- **The flowers and seeds** of many herbs are also edible and high in polyphenols. If your herbs do start to flower or set seed, use these in your recipes as well as the leaves.

- **Some shrubby herbs**, such as rosemary and sage, can become very large over time and may take up too much space in your pot. If this becomes a problem, take cuttings and replace the old plants in the pots in the following growing season.

- **For frost-tender herbs**, such as basil and tarragon, either pot them up and overwinter them inside, or grow more plants from seed the following year. I usually do the latter, often because I want to try new varieties.

- **Dry your herbs** to store and dramatically increase their polyphenol content too. A recent study showed polyphenol levels are maximized by either sun-drying the herbs in a glasshouse or drying them in the oven. To sun-dry, tie the stems with string and hang upside down in a glasshouse or by a sunny window. Or, for even higher polyphenol levels, place herbs on baking sheets in the oven at a very low temperature (about 40°C/105°F) until dry.

PROJECT 6

Polyphenol herb pots

Packed with polyphenols, the disease-preventing phytochemicals that keep us healthy, herbs are easy to grow in pots on a patio or windowsill.

An extremely rich source of phytochemicals, and polyphenols in particular, herbs offer an easy way to increase the diversity in your diet. I love growing them in pots, which I keep close to the kitchen door so that I can easily pop out when cooking and collect a lovely selection.

Most herbs originate from regions with low rainfall, such as the Mediterranean, where they grow wild in nutrient-poor, free-draining soil. This makes them the perfect low-maintenance plants for a patio or balcony. There are some exceptions to this rule, such as many mint species, which come from wetlands or stream-side environments, and basil, a tender plant that originates from tropical zones with relatively high rainfall, but even these do not need much watering.

HERBS FOR POTS

All of these herbs will be happy growing in a pot: thyme, sage, rosemary, mint, lemon balm, oregano, chamomile, parsley, coriander, dill, sorrel, chives, lavender, perilla, basil, chervil and tarragon.

YOU WILL NEED

Large pot (about 45cm/18in wide x 30cm/12in high)

Small pot (about 25cm/10in wide x 20cm/8in high)

Broken clay pieces (crocks)

Potting mix (2:1 ratio of peat-free compost and potting grit)

Gravel topdressing (optional)

Selection of herb plants, such as sage, rosemary, chamomile, thyme and mint

MAKING HERB POTS

1. Place crocks over the drainage holes at the bottom of your pots. Add the potting mix, filling the container to about 10cm/4in from the top. Press the mix down quite firmly to prevent it from sinking too much when wet.

2. Arrange your plants in the pots. Position larger plants, such as rosemary or fennel, to the back or centre of the pot, and lower-growing species, such as thyme, sage or oregano, around the edges.

3. Using a trowel, plant the herbs in your large pot, ensuring they are at the most aesthetically pleasing angle. Firm in well.

4. You can add a layer of gravel over the potting mix around the plants. This helps to prevent the bases of the stems from rotting in damp compost, especially in winter. It also suppresses weed growth and conserves moisture in the summer months by reflecting sunlight.

5. Plant mint in the small pot. Mint is rather invasive and best planted on its own to prevent it swamping its neighbours. Also, because it spreads quickly, it will need repotting regularly, ideally annually, to keep it in good health. In early spring, remove the mint from its pot, divide a section of healthy stems and roots and repot in fresh potting mix.

6. Once planted, water all your herbs in well to help them establish.

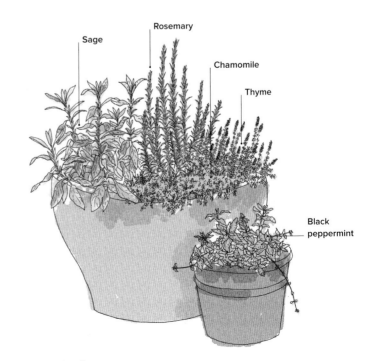

Sage

Rosemary

Chamomile

Thyme

Black peppermint

PROJECT 7

Ferment planters

Where space for crops is limited, try growing the ingredients for some of the delicious ferment recipes in the next chapter in planters on a patio.

If you would like to make your own ferments from home-grown produce but have limited space, try growing your crops in window boxes or planters on a patio or balcony. Here, I've designed a couple of simple containers that will provide the ingredients for a classic sauerkraut (see page 180) and fermented chilli sauce (see page 176). More or less any vegetable or fruit you grow in the garden can be fermented, so feel free to experiment with other edible plants for your pots. The chilli sauce was

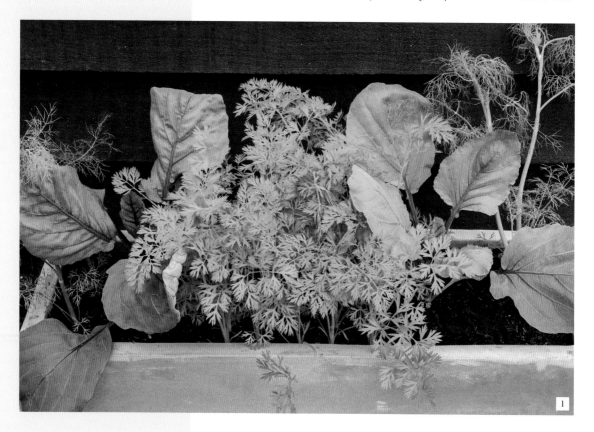

1

a fantastic revelation to me when I started making my own ferments. Its deep, fiery, hot flavour develops during the fermentation process and it makes a fantastic addition to scrambled eggs for breakfast, or use it on any sort of sandwich. Perilla (also known as shiso) is one of my favourite herbs and tastes like a blend between cumin, mint and fennel. The pretty purple leaves are also rich in anthocyanins (see pages 20–21).

Sauerkraut is the classic and most popular fermentation recipe, with good reason. White and red cabbages both lend themselves to fermentation because their crisp, firm texture adds a good bite to the recipe while their mild flavour combines well with the other ingredients.

Making these planters could not be easier and will only take an hour or two at the most. All you will need are the planters, some potting compost and the plants – full instructions are overleaf.

GROWING TIP

Minimize the water you give to your plants to encourage them to accumulate more phytochemicals. Wait until they show some signs of stress and wilt slightly before reaching for the watering can.

1. Make these simple planters to grow the ingredients for sauerkraut and chilli sauce.
2. These crops not only provide you with the ingredients for microbe-rich ferments, they also create a decorative display for a patio, balcony or deep windowsill.

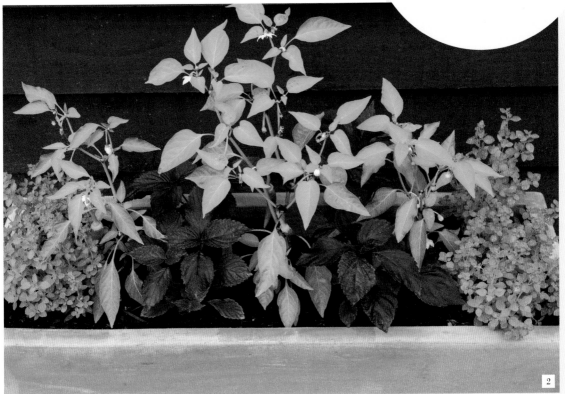

2

YOU WILL NEED

Window boxes or planters
(about 80 x 30 x 30cm/
32 x 12 x 12in)

Potting mix (2:1 ratio of
general-purpose peat-free
compost and potting grit)

Broken terracotta pieces
(crocks)

Organic plant feed, such as a
seaweed feed, compost tea
or fermented plant juice (see
pages 150–51)

Plants for sauerkraut
2 x cabbage plants
(I've used red cabbage
'Cabeza Negra 3')

15–20 x carrot plants
(such as Carrot 'Royal
Chanteray 3')

4–6 x dill plants

Plants for chilli sauce
3 x chilli plants (I've used
Chilli 'Black Hungarian')

4 x small oregano plants

2 x *Perilla frutescens* plants
(such as *Perilla frutescens*
var. *crispa*)

GROW YOUR OWN SAUERKRAUT (see recipe on page 180)

1. Choose white or red cabbage varieties that form tight heads. Sow seed in modules, two seeds per module, in mid-spring, thinning to one seedling when they emerge. Pot on as the plants grow but keep inside.

2. To prepare your planter, place crocks over the drainage holes and fill with potting mix. Press the mix down gently to remove some air pockets, which will prevent it from sinking when watered. Set in a sunny spot.

3. Once the young cabbage plants have developed at least four or five leaves, plant them out in your container using a trowel. Firm them in well. Two or three cabbages should be enough – I've used two here. Cabbages may need protection against cabbage-white butterfly: use a biological control, such as *Bacillus thuringiensis,* or cover with fine mesh.

4. Sow the dill and carrots directly in the container between the cabbages. Sow 2–3 carrot seeds together at 2–3cm/1–1½in spacings and thin to one seedling when they emerge. Thin the dill plants to spacings of 15cm/6in. I often sow dill slightly later in the season, or sow it successively, to give a harvest as the cabbages mature in autumn.

5. Use a seaweed-based feed, compost tea or fermented plant juice to add a microbial and nutrient boost to your plants as they grow.

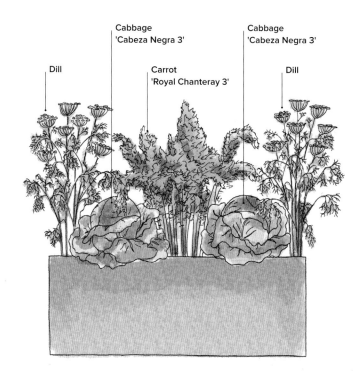

Dill   Cabbage 'Cabeza Negra 3'   Carrot 'Royal Chanteray 3'   Cabbage 'Cabeza Negra 3'   Dill

GROW YOUR OWN FIERY CHILLI FERMENT (see recipe on page 176)

1. Sow the chilli seed in early spring in modules or pots, covering them with a fine layer of vermiculite or compost. Place in a propagator or on a warm windowsill. Seeds should germinate within a couple of weeks at 18–25°C/64–77°F. Pot on the plants when large enough to handle. Remove the stem tips when 15–20cm/6–8in tall to encourage bushy growth and any flowers that develop on the main stem early in the year.

2. To encourage germination, place the perilla seed in a refrigerator for two weeks prior to sowing in mid-spring. Then follow the sowing advice for chillies. Once large enough to handle, transfer them to small pots. Buy oregano plants in spring rather than sowing seed.

3. After the risk of frost has passed, prepare your planter by following the advice in Step 2 for the sauerkraut pot (opposite).

4. Plant your chillies and herbs, allowing space for growth. They will fill out in the pots and you may need to pinch back the stem tips of the perilla to make it more compact and allow space for the other plants.

5. Place your planters in a sunny spot. I feed my plants weekly with organic seaweed, compost tea or fermented plant juice fertilizer. Harvest your chillies in the autumn.

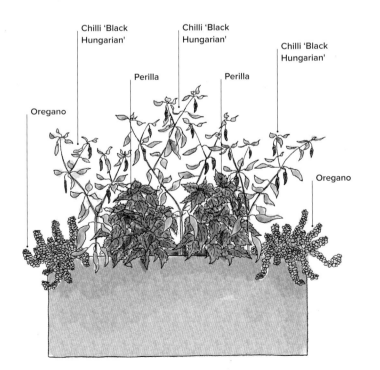

Choosing chilli varieties

With hundreds of varieties of chilli to choose from, consider the following factors when selecting your seeds.

Heat The heat level of chillies is measured in Scoville Heat Units (SHUs) and range from sweet bell peppers with a SHU of zero, up to the crazy, super-hot varieties with 500,000+ SHU. The world's hottest chilli was declared in 2018 to be the infamous 'Carolina Reaper', punching in at an eyeball-popping 2.2 million SHU.

Size Chilli plants vary in size, so check your choices' final heights and spreads before buying. Compact types are best suited to containers and include 'Black Hungarian', 'Fairy Lights', 'Twilight' and 'Stumpy'.

Flavour Chilli flavours vary from fruity to peppery and spicy. One of my favourites for flavour is 'Lemon Drop', which has delicious fruity-flavoured yellow chillies with a good heat – it is too large for a windowsill planter but would be great in a large pot of its own. 'Cherry Bomb' is another personal favourite. It is a perfect size for containers, and has a fantastic spicy heat, without being off the scale. Flavour is very subjective, though, so experiment to see which you like best.

GROWING TIP

Find a really sunny spot to place your planters. Higher levels of sunlight will increase the phytochemical content of your crops. Chilli plants love the sun and heat, so this will also encourage a heavy crop.

PROJECT 8

Food for plant microbes

Use your left-over crops to make these special ferments, which will enrich the soil and your edible plants with beneficial microbes.

Most gardeners will be familiar with the idea of making comfrey or nettle tea to use as liquid fertilizers for their plants. Anyone who's tried them will be familiar with the malodorous stench of rotting foliage in a bucket, and the joy of accidentally slopping it all over yourself as it's decanted into watering cans! While these brews undoubtedly have many benefits, there are alternatives that focus on creating cultures of live bacteria to enrich the plant microbiota – both in the soil and on the surfaces of the plants. This promotes the development of healthier crops, makes nutrients available to the plants, and reduces the risk of foliar diseases.

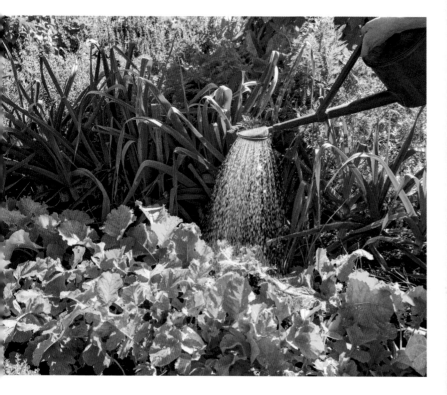

FERMENTED PLANT JUICE: YOU WILL NEED

Approximately 1kg/2lb 3oz of plant material, such as carrots, beetroot, cabbages, carrots, and kale. Include a few different types of plants as they will have different chemical properties.

Approximately 1kg/2lb 3oz molasses (equal weight to the plant material used)

Large bowl and jars

Muslin cloths and rubber bands

COMPOST TEA: YOU WILL NEED

2 x 20–25 litre/5 gallon buckets

1 litre/2 pints of homemade compost

100ml/3.5 fl oz molasses

An aquarium pump

Tea towel or muslin for straining the liquid

Splash of olive oil

Seaweed extract (optional)

FERMENTED PLANT JUICE

This method draws on Korean natural farming techniques. The Koreans have been applying ferments to plants for centuries, and use a wide range of different products, including plant juices. My fermented juice is rich in lactic-acid bacteria, which have a positive effect on plant growth, breaking down organic matter and releasing nutrients into the soil for plants to access. It is difficult to determine exactly which bacteria will be in the juice, and in what quantities. Despite this, the likelihood of building up a rich population of beneficial microbes is very much increased.

1. Chop, shred or roughly blend the plant material and put it into a large bowl.

2. Mix in the molasses thoroughly – avoid refined white sugar, which is less beneficial to the microbes. The molasses provide energy for beneficial bacteria to develop and multiply, enhancing the microbial boost the feed gives your plants.

3. Pack the ingredients into large jars. Seal with fine muslin cloths and rubber bands to prevent insects and debris from entering.

4. Leave the plant feed for 7–14 days to ferment at room temperature and out of direct sunlight. After a few days check for bubbles in the mix – this shows that fermentation is under way.

5. Strain the liquid, which should smell sour, through muslin and bottle and label it. You can also add more molasses before storing the juice. It will keep for months in a refrigerator, but 'burp' the jars periodically so they don't explode as fermentation continues.

Using the plant juice
Dilute the liquid at 2ml per litre/ 0.07fl oz per 2 pints (about one tablespoon in a standard watering can). Use regularly as a foliar feed or soil drench to build up the beneficial microbes.

COMPOST TEA

Compost tea takes the benefits of composting to another level. Use it where access to compost for mulching is limited, as it provides the same microbes in a concentrated form directly to the plants and the rhizosphere (the bioactive area around the plant roots, rich in bacteria and fungi). Compost is brewed in water, together with a source of nutrients for the microbes to ferment, such as molasses or seaweed (or both). Air is then pumped into the mix to provide oxygen for the microbes.

1. If using mains water, pour it into a bucket, insert the aquarium pump and turn on for a couple of hours prior to adding the rest of your ingredients. This should dissipate the chlorine in the water, which may have a negative impact on the microbes.

2. Put your home-made compost into a bucket and top up with the de-chlorinated water. Leave at least 10cm/4in at the top of the bucket so you can stir the mix without it spilling over the edges.

3. Stir in the molasses so they are thoroughly distributed throughout the mix. You can also add some seaweed extract to the tea now; 10–20ml/0.35–0.7fl oz should be sufficient to help kickstart the fermentation process.

4. Add a splash of olive oil to the compost tea, which stops the mix bubbling over the top of the bucket as it brews.

5. Insert the pump and switch it on. Stir the tea once or twice a day to make sure it is well aerated throughout.

6. Leave your tea for three days to ferment, then strain it into a second bucket, using the tea towel or muslin.

Using the compost tea
Use a sprayer to apply the tea as a foliage feed on to your plants or pour it into a watering can and use as a soil drench around the root zone to increase the richness and diversity of the plant microbiota (see pages 26–27).

PROJECT 9

Sprouting seeds

Easy to make at home, sprouts' exceptionally high levels of phytochemicals and antioxidants help to prevent cancer, diabetes and other diseases.

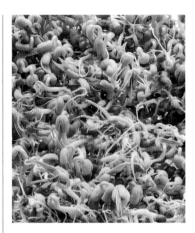

Sprouting seeds may not spring to mind when you think of traditional grow-your-own projects. It is a horticultural practice, though, as the seeds germinate and the resulting plants are harvested, just at a very immature stage. Sprouts, or microgreens, are amazingly good for us. They are five to ten times richer in nutrients than the mature plants. This means we only need to eat a small portion of these nutrient bombs to gain the same health benefits as from a fully grown plant.

Significant increases in polyphenols, flavonols and antioxidant activity (see pages 20–21) have been found in the sprouted seeds of many vegetables, fruits and flowers, including soybeans, chickpeas, mung beans, buckwheat, sunflowers, broccoli, radishes and fenugreek. For example, radish sprouts have been found to have nearly seven times the polyphenol content of the mature roots, while three-day-old sprouts of broccoli and cauliflower have 10–100 times as much glucosinolates (see page 71), with their multiple health benefits, compared to mature florets.

How seeds sprout into superfoods

Research shows that you can increase levels of vitamins, glucosinolates and other polyphenols in sprouts to an even higher degree by using 'elicitors'. These are substances or conditions that cause physical changes in the plants, such as exposing the sprouts to high levels of sunlight, putting them in cold conditions, or adding salt. Seaweed feed also raises polyphenol levels.

Lots of chemical changes are triggered when seeds germinate, which boost their health benefits. The seed stores energy in the form of protein, fat and carbohydrates, which are broken down during germination and converted to meet the nutritional needs of the young plant.

As the seeds germinate, phytochemicals also increase to help defend the vulnerable seedlings from damage and ensure that they grow into healthy mature plants.

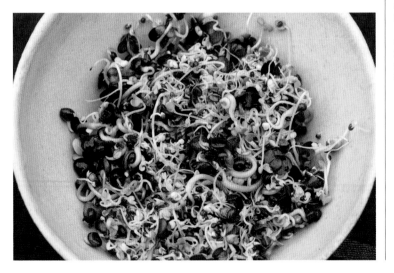

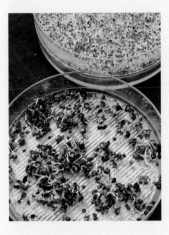

YOU WILL NEED

Seed sprouter or a wide-mouthed jar with a mesh or muslin cover and rubber band

Seeds of your choice

SEEDS TO SPROUT

These seeds are perfect for sprouting and will germinate in 3–7 days: kale, alfalfa, red cabbages, broccoli, peas, red clover, lentils, radishes, soybeans, chickpeas, mung beans, buckwheat, sunflowers, broccoli and fenugreek.

HOW TO MAKE SPROUTS

1. Make sure the seeds you use for sprouting haven't been processed and use whole seeds, not grains that are described as having been rolled, hulled or pearled.

2. If using a jar, simply place your seeds in it. How many seeds you include really depends on the type, but adding them to a depth of 2cm/1in in the base of the jar should be fine.

3. Cover with plenty of water, seal with the muslin or mesh cover, and soak overnight.

4. Drain the jar through the muslin the following morning and leave it on its side, out of direct sunlight at room temperature. Cover again with water and rinse and drain the seeds 2–3 times a day.

5. If using a sprouter with different levels, it's even easier. Distribute your seeds thinly on each layer. Top up with water and allow it to drain through to the base, then pour out the water that has collected in the bottom tray. Repeat 2–3 times a day.

6. Your seeds should be fully sprouted in approximately 3–7 days, depending on the variety. You can then use them immediately or seal them in a bag and store in the refrigerator; they will keep for a few days.

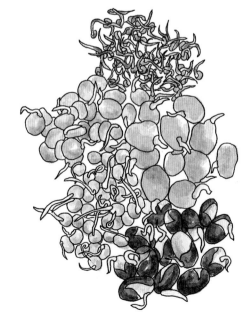

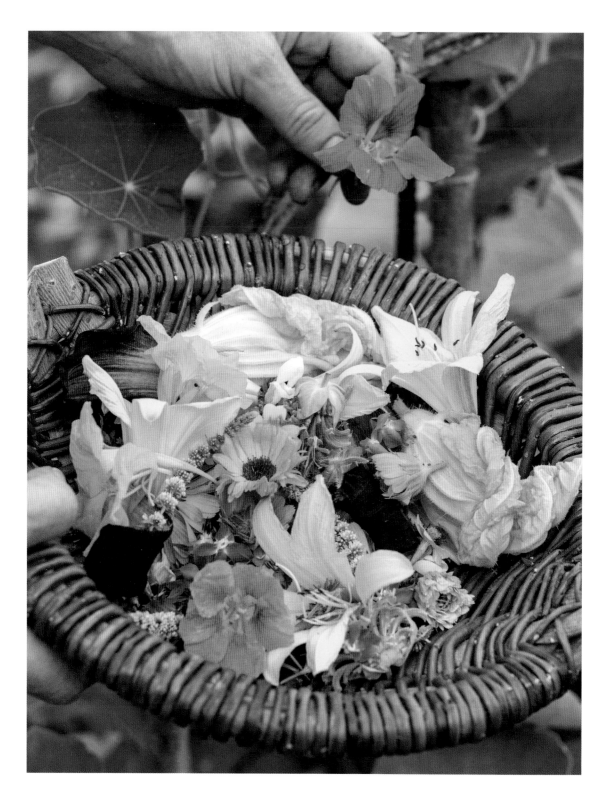

PROJECT 10

Edible flowers

Flowers that we can eat have huge benefits for our gut microbiota. Use the blooms as garnishes, batter and stir-fry them, or bake them in biscuits.

Edible flowers are a beautiful addition to any meal, and they are highly beneficial from a nutritional point of view, boosting the diversity of beneficial microbes in the gut. Difficult to store and transport, you rarely find them for sale in the shops, yet most are very easy to grow at home.

The nutritional benefits of flowers come from the pollen, nectar and the petals. Edible flowers contain high levels of phytochemicals, especially polyphenols, which determine their colour and scent, so they can attract pollinators. These compounds keep the flowers in good condition for longer, too, allowing time for pollination to occur. There is a strong correlation between phytochemical content and antioxidant activity, which also has tremendous health benefits.

The types of phytochemical you will find in edible flowers depends on the plant species and the variety. The most important compounds are flavonoids and carotenoids (see pages 20–21) and, as a general rule, flowers with darker colours have higher levels of these phytochemicals and greater antioxidant activity. However, white elderflowers are extremely rich sources of quercetin and rutin, which strengthen cardiovascular health, protect against cancer and reduce inflammation. The phytochemical levels in elderflowers are, in fact, higher than in most edible flowers, so do not dismiss them and try to eat a range of hues.

Some flowers we can eat have particularly high levels of polyphenols. For example, in a study of 65 edible flowers, *Rosa rugosa* came out top, with 55 times higher levels of polyphenols than cucumber flowers. As always, the key is diversity and to help you I have selected ten lovely flowers (overleaf) for you to grow and enjoy in multi-ingredient meals.

HARVESTING TIPS

- Select disease-free and undamaged flowers.
- Harvest the flowers at cool times of the day and when they are in full bloom.
- Remove the base of the flower (the calyx) if the texture is disagreeable.
- Use the flowers shortly after picking. Store them in a cool place and pop the flower stems in a glass of water to keep them fresh.
- Blow on the flowers before harvesting to remove any insects that may be hiding inside.

Left *Collect a basket of colourful edible flowers from the flower and vegetable garden, such as nasturtiums, marigolds, daylilies, courgette and borage blooms.*

Ten easy edible flowers to grow

Here are some of my favourite edible flowers. All are easy to grow, rich in a wide range of phytochemicals, and add colour to any meal.

1 Rose
(*Rosa rugosa/Rosa davurica*)

Growing tips Grow these shrub roses in a sunny spot. Remove dead and damaged stems, and shorten the flowering stems by a third from late autumn to late winter.

Flower uses Roses have a slightly sweet, perfumed flavour. Freeze the petals in ice cubes or add them to teas and use as garnishes for desserts.

2 Nasturtium
(*Tropaeolum* species)

Growing tips Sow seed in spring outside or inside in small pots. Cut plants back hard in midsummer for a longer flowering period.

Flower uses Use the blooms' peppery flavour to spice up salads or as garnishes for savoury dishes.

3 Chrysanthemum
(*Chrysanthemum* species)

Growing tips These perennials tolerate temperatures down to -5°C/23°F and need full sun to flower. Lift and protect plants inside in winter.

Flower uses The mild-flavoured blooms make a decorative garnish for savoury dishes and desserts.

4 French marigold
(*Tagetes patula*)

Growing tips Sow annually in modules inside and plant out after the frosts. Pinch out the growing tips for bushier growth.

Flower uses Use the spicy flowers to make teas or as a garnish on savoury dishes.

5 Daylily
(*Hemerocallis* species)

Growing tips These perennials grow back year after year. Grow them in sun or part-shade and reasonably fertile soil. Cut back old foliage in winter or early spring.

Flower uses Daylilies have a mild flavour, similar to a courgette. Use as a garnish on savoury dishes and salads or even on desserts. *Hemerocallis lilioasphodelus* is a particularly good species to use.

6 Elder
(*Sambucus nigra*)

Growing tips Prune this large shrub back hard over winter, removing old, dead and damaged growth. It will be happy in sun or part shade.

Flower uses Use the sweet flowers to make elderflower champagne or cordial.

7 Cornflower
(*Centaurea cyanus*)

Growing tips Sow the seed of this annual outside in a sunny spot in mid-spring.

Flower uses The spicy, blue flowers make a lovely garnish for savoury dishes and salads.

8 Violets
(*Viola tricolor/Viola odorata*)

Growing tips In spring, sow the seed indoors in modules or outside in either a sunny or partially shaded area.

Flower uses The mild-flavoured flowers make pretty garnishes for savoury dishes, desserts, cakes and biscuits.

9 Pinks
(*Dianthus* species)

Growing tips These hardy perennials will bloom year after year in a sunny spot and free-draining soil. The German pink (*Dianthus carthusianorum*) is a good edible choice and looks beautiful in a herbaceous border.

Flower uses The clove-flavoured flowers make a good accompaniment to spicy dishes or desserts.

10 Japanese honeysuckle
(*Lonicera japonica*)

Growing tips Grow this vigorous, hardy climbing plant in sun or part-shade and prune hard in early spring.

Flower uses The sweet, honey-flavoured flowers can be used to make tea infusions or to garnish desserts and cakes.

WORDS OF WARNING

- Always make sure the flowers you are harvesting are edible and not toxic – reputable horticulture websites offer guides. Choose plants that you've either grown yourself from seed you know the provenance of, or from plants that are clearly labelled when you buy them.
- Avoid foraging roadside flowers that might be contaminated with particulates from traffic or pesticides from nearby farms.
- Avoid using flowers from the florist, unless you know they haven't been preserved with chemicals with toxicity warnings.

EDIBLE FLOWERS TO TRY

Choose from the following flowers to grow to eat: *Rosa rugosa* (top left), honeysuckle (top right), cornflower (bottom right) and daylily (bottom left). Other flowers to try include salvia, borage, lavender, courgette, chicory, rosemary, hibiscus, osmanthus and malva.

HARVESTING TIP

Harvest your seeds on a dry day, at the point when they would naturally disperse. This is often as the pods or capsules start to open, or the seeds darken in colour.

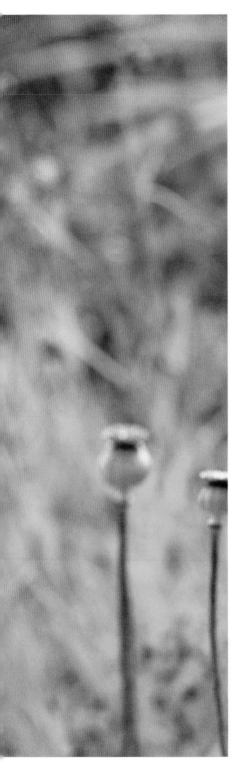

PROJECT 11

Edible seeds

Rich sources of phytochemicals, edible seeds pack a punch nutritionally and add depth to the flavour of bread, cakes and almost any savoury dish.

Growing seeds to add to a plant-based diet enriches it with a range of phytochemicals, especially polyphenols, and they offer one of the best ways to nourish your gut microbes. Seeds are a versatile source of phytochemicals in concentrated form and including them in our meals or as snacks helps to increase the diversity in our diets. They are also a fantastic source of fibre, healthy fats, vitamins and minerals. Sprinkle your home-grown seeds on salads, porridge and sandwiches, or add them to the cooking pot.

It used to bother me when herbs and vegetables bolted and started flowering in the edible garden. Now I see it as an opportunity to harvest different parts of the plant that will be high in nutritional value. Phytochemicals accumulate in the flowers and seeds of plants once they reach maturity and are ready to reproduce. They help to preserve the seeds, protecting them from deteriorating too quickly, before they have had the chance to germinate. They are often different to those found in other parts of the plant, too, and are extremely good for our gut microbiota (see pages 16–19) and our overall health.

There are lots of plants you can grow for their seeds in the edible garden. Some traditional vegetable crops, such as peas, beans and other legumes, are seeds themselves of course, but in this project I've focused on a few of the more unusual plants you can grow (see overleaf). All of their seeds are nutritious and the herbs, in particular, are especially high in polyphenols (see pages 20–21).

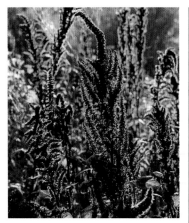

Amaranth

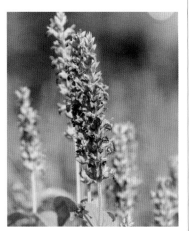

Chia

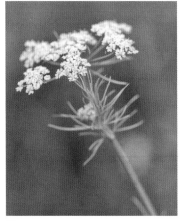

Caraway

Best plants to grow for seed

These plants' seeds are rich sources of fibre, fats, protein, vitamins, minerals and phytochemicals. They also contain tocopherols, a type of vitamin E with potent antioxidant properties that strengthens the immune system.

Quinoa and Amaranth

Quinoa and amaranth (*Chenopodium quinoa* and *Amaranthus*) are often heralded as superfoods for their high levels of protein, omega-3 fatty acids, vitamins and minerals. They also contain lots of phytochemicals, including betalains (most commonly found in beetroot), carotenoids (see pages 20–21) and tocopherols, a form of vitamin E. Scientific studies have associated tocopherols with a reduction in heart disease, a delay in the onset of Alzheimer's disease and cancer prevention.

Growing advice Sow the seed in early spring indoors, or outside from late spring after the risk of frost has passed. Space plants approximately 40cm/16in apart. You may need to protect young plants from pigeon attacks with bird-proof mesh.

Harvesting The seeds are ready to harvest when you see them about to fall from the plant. Remove the chaff (seed coverings) from the seed using a fine sieve and store in an airtight container in a cool, dark place.

Chia

The seeds of this annual sage, known as chia (*Salvia hispanica*), are powerhouses of nutrition, packing in very high levels of omega-3 fatty acids, protein and fibre, which is good news for our gut microbes. They also have very high levels of polyphenols and excellent antioxidant activity.

Growing advice Sow seed from early to late spring indoors. After the risk of frosts has passed, plant outside approximately 60cm/24in apart – these large plants can grow up to 2m/7ft high.

Harvesting Harvest the seeds at the point of natural dispersal. Remove the chaff (seed coverings) with a sieve and store the seeds in an airtight container.

Fennel

Fennel seeds (*Foeniculum vulgare*) are a great source of polyphenols with high antioxidant activity and studies show that they are useful as antibacterial agents too. In fact, the food industry is testing fennel seeds as a preservative, to inhibit the growth of dangerous bacteria.

Growing advice Sow fennel seed in a sunny spot outside, thinning once it germinates to about 40cm/16in apart. Plants are perennial, appearing year after year – cut back the old foliage in early spring. Fennel self-seeds everywhere so remove unwanted seedlings in spring.

Harvesting Remove the seed heads at the point of natural dispersal and store in an airtight container in a cool place.

Radish

The seeds of radishes (*Raphanus sativus*) are rich in glucosinolates, which have important cancer prevention properties. The radish cultivar 'Rat's Tail' is grown specifically for its edible seed pods.

Growing advice Sow seed directly outside from mid-spring until late summer. Sow thinly, allowing an eventual spacing between plants of approximately 15cm/6in.

Harvesting Eat the seed pods when they are young and tender.

Poppy

Poppy flowers (*Papaver* species) produce a vast number of seeds, which are highly valued for their antioxidant activity. Poppy seeds are also rich in flavonoids and tocopherols (see Quinoa and Amaranth).

Growing advice Sow seed in early spring indoors, and transplant seedlings into modules as they grow. Plant outside in late spring, about 20–30cm/8–12in apart. Alternatively, sow seed directly outside in late spring.

Harvesting Wait until the seed capsules are dry and the top is open, indicating that the seeds are ready to disperse. Either break the capsules open to reveal the seeds or shake them out into an airtight container. Store in a cool place.

Nigella

Known as love-in-a-mist, nigella (*Nigella damascena*) flowers make beautiful garden plants and will self-seed everywhere, given the chance. They contain tocopherols (see Quinoa and Amaranth), flavonoids, and several active compounds that help to protect against diseases, including Alzheimer's and Parkinson's.

Growing advice Sow seed indoors in early spring and transplant the seedlings into modules as they grow. Plant outside in a sunny spot and well-drained soil from mid- to late spring, about 20–25cm/8–10in apart. Alternatively, plant the seed directly outside in autumn or early spring.

Harvesting Wait until the seed capsules are dry, indicating that they are ready to disperse. Break the capsule open to reveal the seeds and shake out into an airtight container, removing any chaff (seed coating) before sealing it. Store in a cool place.

Pumpkin

There's probably no point growing pumpkins (*Cucurbita* species) for their seeds alone, but when you harvest them, eat the seeds for an extra source of nutrition. Packed with a variety of different phytochemicals to the fruit, the seeds contain tocopherols (see Quinoa and Amaranth) and have good antioxidant properties. Studies show the seeds of *Cucurbita pepo* have higher phytochemical levels than those of *Cucurbita maxima*.

Growing advice Sow seed in mid-spring indoors and plant outside after the frosts, in late spring or early summer. Pumpkin plants are sprawling and need lots of space to grow so allow at least 1m/3ft between plants.

Harvesting Harvest the fruits in autumn, once fully matured. Slice them open and spoon out the seeds, wash to remove any pulp, and spread them out on a baking tray or other surface to dry. Make sure they're not layered on top of each other – good airflow will prevent them from rotting. They may take a few weeks to dry properly, after which they can be stored in an airtight container somewhere cool and dry. They are delicious roasted or pan-fried.

Caraway

Studies show that caraway seeds (*Carum carvi*) have over four times the total amount of phytochemicals of other herbs and spices, such as turmeric, dill, marjoram and nutmeg. The plants are easy to grow and before they set seed, caraway also produces pretty flowers that look great, especially in a meadow-style scheme.

Growing advice Sow seed indoors from early to mid-spring and transplant the seedlings into modules, before planting outside from late spring onwards.

Harvesting Harvest the whole seed heads of the plant at the point of natural dispersal. Remove the seed from the heads and discard any chaff (seed coating). Store in an airtight container in a cool place.

Lovage

Studies show that seeds of the lovage plant (*Levisticum officinale*) contain the highest source of polyphenols, compared to the leaves, roots and stems. This perennial plant comes back each year, dying down during the winter months and emerging again in spring, and needs little care and attention once it is established.

Growing advice Lovage is a large plant, growing up to 2m/7ft in height, so make sure you have plenty of space for it. You probably only need one plant, especially because the seeds have a very strong flavour and are only used in small quantities. Grow from seed sown in early to mid-spring indoors, and plant out in late spring, or buy a young plant to grow on. Cut back the old foliage in early spring.

Harvesting Remove the seed heads at the point of natural dispersal. Store the seeds in an airtight container in a cool place.

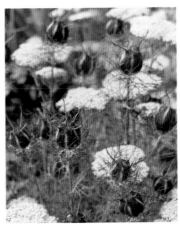

Nigella

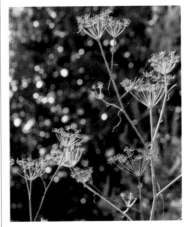

Fennel

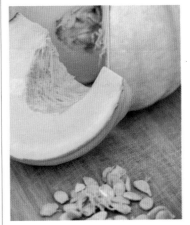

Pumpkin

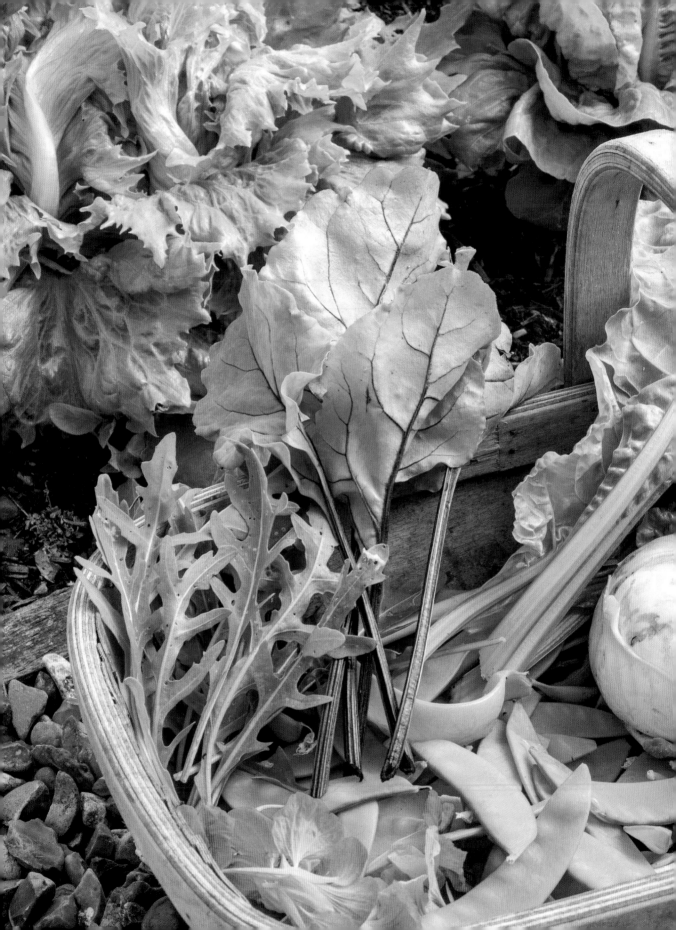

CHAPTER FOUR

Ferment Recipes

"Try these delicious recipes to make the most of your home-grown crops and to give your gut a boost of beneficial microbes."

Fermenting for gut health

This simple method of preserving food has been used for centuries, and we now know that fermenting is not only a great way to enjoy our home-grown crops, it's also exceptionally good for our health.

Fermentation is a traditional preservation technique and many fermented foods, such as bread, cheese, olives and yoghurt, may already be a familiar part of your diet. Other more exotic-sounding ferments, including kimchi, sauerkraut, kombucha and kefir, are becoming increasingly popular as we learn more about their benefits for gut health and our microbiota. Fermentation sounds complicated, but it is extremely easy to do at home with the vegetables, herbs and fruit you've grown in the garden.

The type of fermentation I have used to preserve the garden produce in the recipes in this chapter is called lactic acid fermentation. In this process the vegetables are submerged in a salty brine that prevents them from being exposed to harmful bacteria. Microbes that naturally exist on the plants then set to work, breaking down carbohydrates, such as the sugars, in the food and converting them into lactic acid. It is this acid that is responsible for preserving the vegetables and transforming the flavour, giving the ferments a deliciously sour tang.

In the following pages, I've outlined some basic recipes using seasonal crops, with some simple instructions to get you started. You can then use the same methods with other produce you have to hand to make ferments tailored to the specific crops you are growing. When thinking about what combinations to use, I experiment by combining the ingredients that work well together in my favourite dishes and play with them to devise my own ferment recipes.

Fermentation tips

How much salt?
You can change the quantities of produce I've used in the recipes in this chapter, but you will then need to recalculate how much salt to add to them. For every 100g/3.5oz of produce, you will require 2–3g/ 0.07–0.1oz of unrefined sea salt. So, for example, if you have 1kg/35oz of sliced cabbage and carrot to ferment, you will need to add 1½–2 tablespoons of salt.

Fermentation times
The time it takes for produce to ferment depends on temperature. In warmer conditions, the process will be quicker. After the first few days, taste the ferment every day or two until it reaches the degree of sourness you prefer. Once you have gained a little experience, you will be able to judge more easily when the ferment is ready. The fermentation process does not end when it's in the refrigerator either – cold temperatures simply slow it down and you will find the flavours continue to evolve over time.

Storage times
I never manage to keep my ferments for very long before eating them, but they should last for at least three months in a refrigerator.

EQUIPMENT YOU WILL NEED

Some fermentation recipes may call for different equipment, but these items, together with bowls, knives and a chopping board, work well for me.

1. Wide-mouthed mason jars with lids
The wide mouths of these glass jars make it easier to pack in the ingredients tightly.

2. Airlock
These are essentially one-way valves that allow carbon dioxide to escape from the jars during fermentation, while ensuring oxygen cannot enter, thereby preventing the ferment from spoiling.

3. Glass weights
Use these weights to submerge the ingredients under the brine. The liquid creates an oxygen-free environment that prevents the ferments from rotting.

4. Mandolin
Useful for slicing vegetables very finely, a mandolin increases the surface area of the produce, allowing salt to quickly penetrate into it. This tool also helps to create ferments with a great texture.

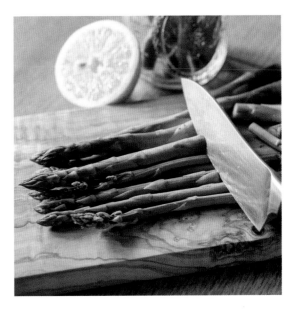

5. Wooden tamper
Use the tamper to pack the ingredients tightly into the mason jars.

6. Scales
Electric scales are best because they allow you to measure out precise quantities.

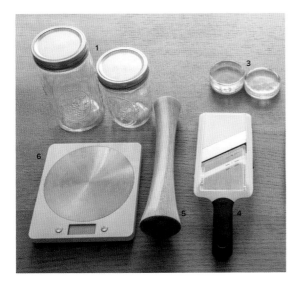

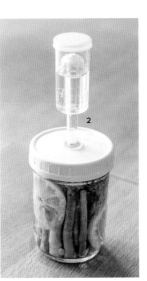

Above *Freshly harvested crops tend to have a higher moisture content than supermarket-bought produce, which means the ferments quickly develop a liquid brine.*

Spring & early summer recipes

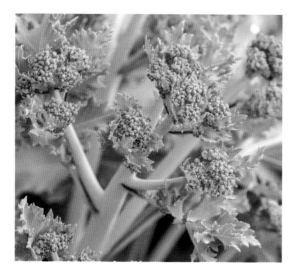

SEAKALE WITH CHICORY, DILL AND LEMON

Seakale is so evocative of the coast. Harvesting the leaves immediately conjures up images for me of the shingle beaches where it grows, battling against the elements. It's an easy-going perennial that will thrive in most soil types. The plants are usually bought as thongs (root cuttings), which you plant out in early spring and they will then quickly establish during the first year of growth. Seakale is a wonderful plant to use in fermentation recipes, retaining its dark iron-rich flavour. In this recipe I've added chicory, dill and lemon to add layers of bitterness and sharpness.

Ingredients

1.5kg/3lb 5oz seakale
500g/1lb 2oz chicory
3 tbsp unrefined sea salt
1 lemon (juice and zest)
Large handful of dill (chopped)

Method

1. Thinly slice the seakale and chicory. I used a mandolin for the chicory to create a fine texture.

2. Rub in the unrefined sea salt thoroughly. You will find the seakale will reduce drastically in bulk because it has such a high water content, which the salting process removes.

3. Stir in the juice and zest of the lemon, and the dill.

4. Pack all your ingredients tightly into mason jars. Place glass weights on the surface to submerge the ingredients under the brine before sealing the jars with an airlock (see page 165).

5. Leave to ferment at room temperature for 5–7 days or until the ferment has developed the degree of sourness you desire.

6. Remove the airlock, seal the jars with their lids and store in the refrigerator. This ferment should then keep for at least a few months.

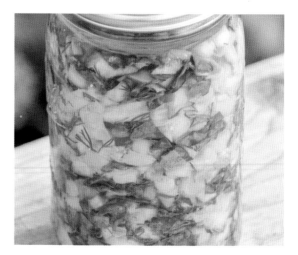

FENNEL, ASPARAGUS AND ORANGE PICKLE

Last spring I made the family fennel, asparagus and orange salad, and we enjoyed it so much I decided to try the combination in ferment form. It works really well – you can still taste all the flavours, with a fermented tangy edge. Asparagus is so delicious eaten fresh, I find it difficult to save any for preserving, but at least this way we can enjoy it for longer.

Ingredients

400g/14oz Florence fennel bulbs
  (about 2 bulbs)
800g/1lb 12oz cabbage (about one head)
300g/10oz asparagus spears
2 tbsp unrefined sea salt
1 orange (juice and zest)

"The blend of sweet and savoury flavours in this fruity pickle goes brilliantly with salads and cheese."

Method

1. Slice the Florence fennel and cabbage very finely. A mandolin offers the quickest way to do this.

2. Slice the asparagus spears into small chunks.

3. Rub the salt into the sliced vegetables thoroughly until they are glistening with moisture.

4. Stir in the orange juice and zest.

5. Pack all the ingredients tightly into mason jars with a tamper. Submerge the ingredients under the brine with a glass weight and seal with an airlock (see page 165).

6. Leave to ferment at room temperature for approximately 5–7 days or until you are happy with the sourness of the flavour.

7. Remove the airlock, seal with the jar lid and store in a cool place. It will keep in the refrigerator for at least three months.

SPICY SUMAC KOHLRABI

If you've not tried sumac before, give it a go – it has a really interesting taste. Produced from the ground berries of the shrub *Rhus typhina* (stag's horn sumac), the flavour is best described as tangy and citrusy. I buy the powder but it would be possible to make your own if you have a sumac in the garden. This is easily done by grinding the berries in a blender and sifting the red powder from the seed to use as a spice. The combination of sumac and the Korean spice gochugaru gives this dish a wonderful chilli kick, without being overpowering. Most of my tasters agree that this is one of my best ferments.

At first, I found that this spicy ferment had a taste distinctly reminiscent of Frazzle crisps, but don't be deterred – the flavour soon develops and the tingly frazzliness then disappears.

Ingredients

1kg/2lb 3oz) kohlrabi
1½ tbsp unrefined sea salt
½ tbsp sumac powder
1 tbsp gochugaru (Korean red pepper flakes)
  or chilli flakes

Method

1. Slice the kohlrabi thinly – I used a mandolin for this – then chop it into strips.

2. Rub the sea salt into the sliced kohlrabi. The salt causes moisture to be released from the vegetables which creates a brine.

3. Stir in the sumac powder and gochugaru (or chilli flakes).

4. Pack the ingredients tightly into wide-mouthed mason jars using a tamper and submerge the ferment under the brine with a glass weight.

5. Seal the ferment with an airlock (see page 165) and leave for 5–7 days at room temperature, or until the ferments have achieved the preferred level of sourness.

6. Remove the airlock and seal the jar with its lid. This ferment should store in the refrigerator for at least three months.

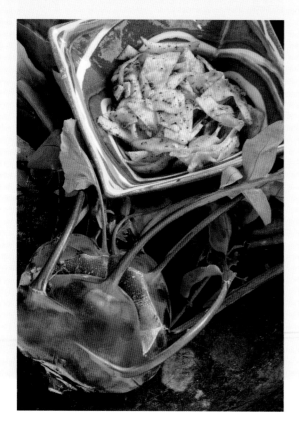

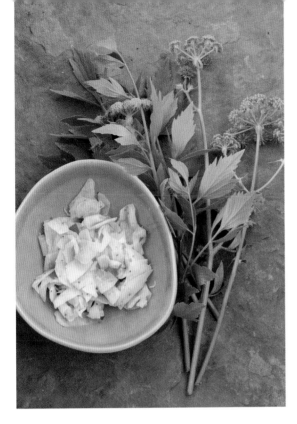

KOHLRABI WITH LOVAGE AND CELERY SEED

The crunchy texture of kohlrabi is retained during fermentation and its mild taste is an excellent foundation to layer with other ingredients. Lovage and celery are strong flavours but used in moderation give a wonderful savoury complexity. This is a sophisticated ferment and an excellent companion to any sort of cheese dish.

Ingredients

1kg/2lb3oz kohlrabi
1½ tbsp unrefined sea salt
1 tbsp celery seeds
1 handful of lovage leaves, chopped
Small lemon (juice and zest)

Method

1. Slice the kohlrabi thinly using a mandolin, then chop it into strips.

2. Rub the sea salt into the sliced kohlrabi thoroughly. The salt causes moisture to be released from the vegetables which creates a brine.

3. Mix in the celery seeds, chopped lovage leaves and the zest and juice of the lemon.

4. Pack the kohlrabi mixture into jars – wide-mouthed mason jars are ideal. Weigh down your mixture with a glass weight to ensure the mixture remains submerged under the brine.

5. Seal the ferment with an airlock (see page 165) and leave for approximately 5–7 days at room temperature, or until the ferments have achieved the level of sourness you desire.

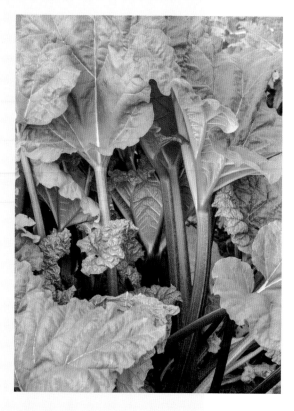

RHUBARB KOMBUCHA

Kombucha is a delicious, refreshing fizzy drink made from fermented tea and, as I'm an obsessive tea drinker, it is naturally my probiotic drink of choice. The tea is fermented with a kombucha culture of bacteria and yeast, which creates a beverage teaming with microbes. Rapidly gaining popularity in shops and restaurants, kombucha can be expensive to buy, but it's very easy to make at home at a fraction of the price. You can also flavour it with infusions of fruits and herbs from your edible garden and this recipe for rhubarb kombucha is my absolute favourite. Try my method first, and then experiment with other crops to find your favourite brew.

Ingredients for the brew

6–8 teabags (or 3–4 teaspoons of loose tea with
  a tea infuser). It is your choice whether to use black,
  green or white tea – I prefer white tea for its subtle
  flavour. Do not use fruit or herbal teas.
170g/6oz granulated sugar for the kombucha
Kombucha culture (or scoby), which is a starter culture
  of live yeast and bacteria. You can buy a scoby
  online to get you started.

Ingredients for the rhubarb infusion

500g/1lb 2oz rhubarb stems (leaves removed
  as these are poisonous)
100g/3½oz caster sugar
2 tbsp water

This ferment is also delicious with the addition of sweet cicely (*Myrrhis odorata*), which gives the kombucha a hint of sweet aniseed flavour.

YOU WILL NEED

Large heat-proof bowl/container
(for the sweet tea to brew in)

2.5l/4½pt glass jar/container

Muslin cloth and rubber band
to cover the top of the jar

Small heat-proof bowl

Saucepan

Sieve

2l/4pt boiled water

2 x 1l/2pt swing-top
glass bottles

Method

Stage 1: Making the brew

1. Put the teabags or loose leaf tea (ideally in a loose leaf tea infuser) in the heat-proof bowl and add the granulated sugar and boiled water. Stir well.

2. Allow your tea to brew for 20–30 minutes, then remove the tea and leave it to cool.

3. Once the tea is cool to the touch, transfer it to the large 2.5-litre/4½pint jar.

4. Add the scoby to the jar (lightest side upwards) and add about 125ml/4 fl oz of the starter liquid that will have been delivered with your scoby (or retained from your last brew).

5. Cover the jar with the muslin cloth and wait for it to brew. This usually takes between 7–-10 days but you can leave if for longer if you prefer a sourer flavour.

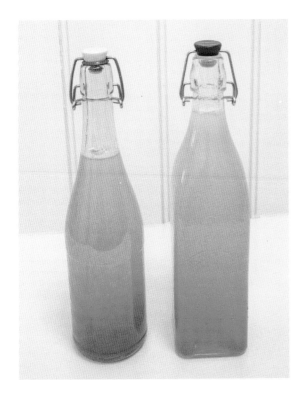

Stage 2: The second fermentation

1. After the kombucha has finished the first stage of fermentation, prepare your rhubarb infusion. Roughly chop the rhubarb and add to a saucepan with the sugar and water.

2. Bring to the boil and simmer for 10–15 minutes, or until the rhubarb is soft and there is plenty of liquid in the pan.

3. Strain the liquid into a heat-proof bowl using the sieve and put to one side to cool. This is the rhubarb infusion you will be adding to your kombucha later. Use the remaining stewed rhubarb however you fancy – I like mine on yoghurt or cereal.

4. Pour your kombucha into the glass bottles, reserving approximately 125ml/4fl oz of the liquid as a starter for your next brew. Leave enough room at the top of the bottles to pour in your rhubarb infusion.

5. Add the rhubarb infusion and seal the bottles. Leave to ferment for a second time at room temperature for 1–3 days. This is when your kombucha will get fizzy. 'Burp' your bottles daily to avoid a build-up of gas and a kombucha explosion!

6. The kombucha can be stored in the refrigerator for a few months. The fermentation process will continue in cold storage so burp your bottles now and again.

> "Flavour your kombucha drinks with home-grown fruits or herbs from the garden."

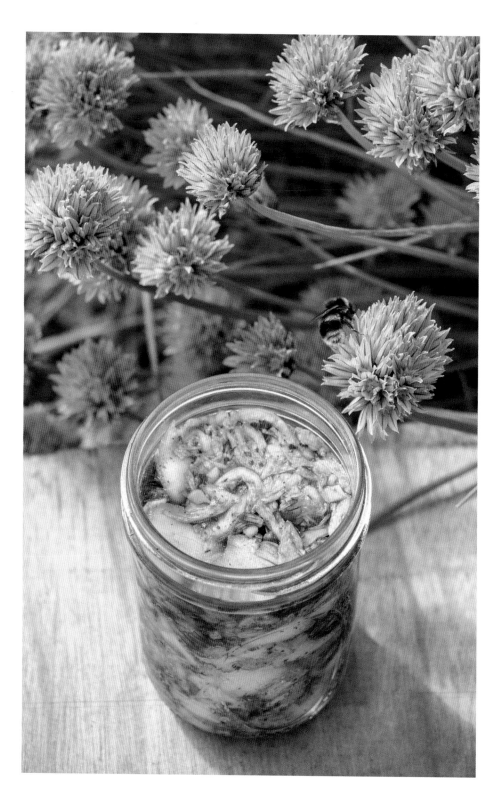

Midsummer recipes

KIMCHI WITH CHIVE FLOWERS

No set of fermentation recipes would be complete without kimchi. Traditional recipes usually include fish sauce, but mine is vegan and I have used soy sauce instead, which I don't think in any way compromises the flavour when combined with the fresh garden ingredients. Many recipes also use spring onions, but I've substituted these for chive flowers. The blooms have a similar oniony flavour, but add an interesting texture and look really pretty.

Method

1. Remove their stems, then chop the Chinese cabbages into small chunks.

2. Place the cabbage in a large bowl and rub in the sea salt thoroughly. The cabbage will quickly start releasing moisture. Cover it with a plate to keep it submerged under the brine and leave it for about eight hours (or overnight).

3. Rinse the cabbage thoroughly and leave to drain.

4. Chop and crush the ginger and garlic. Mix in the soy sauce, gochugaru and sugar. I used a pestle and mortar to crush the garlic and ginger, but you could just use a blender.

5. Add the chive flowers and mix all the ingredients together in a large bowl.

6. Pack the ingredients into wide-mouthed mason jars. Place glass weights on the top to keep the fermented ingredients submerged under the brine.

7. Seal the jars with airlocks (see page 165) and leave for 3–5 days. Kimchi is usually slightly quicker to ferment than some other ferments. Taste regularly until it reaches the desired level of fiery pickliness.

Ingredients

2 Chinese cabbages
4 tbsp unrefined sea salt
2cm/1in piece of ginger
5 garlic cloves
2 tbsp soy sauce
1–2 tbsp gochugaru (Korean red pepper flakes) or chilli flakes
2 tsp caster sugar
30–40 chive flowers

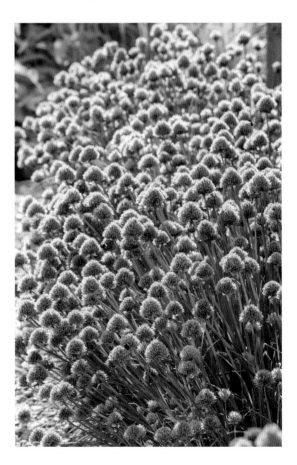

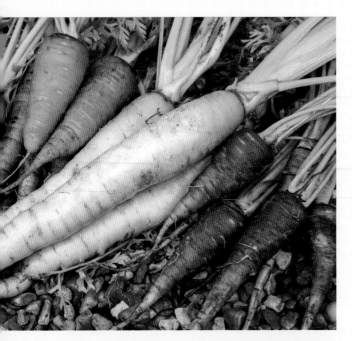

BEETROOT, CARROT AND CARAWAY PICKLE

Caraway seeds are an excellent ingredient to add to ferments. Traditionally used in sauerkraut, in this recipe the seeds' mild peppery aniseed flavour works as a subtle contrast to the sweet beetroot and carrot. I've found this ferment is a great accompaniment to smoked fish dishes.

Ingredients

750g/1lb 10oz beetroot
750g/1lb 10oz carrot
2 tbsp unrefined sea salt
1 tbsp caraway seeds

Method

1. Finely slice the beetroot and carrot. I use a mandolin to ensure the slices are very thin.

2. Rub the unrefined sea salt into the vegetables thoroughly, which will release the water in them to make a brine.

3. Stir in the caraway seeds.

4. Pack the ingredients tightly into mason jars. Submerge the vegetables under the brine using glass weights, then seal each jar with an airlock (see page 165).

5. Leave to ferment at room temperature for 5–7 days or until it reaches your preferred degree of sourness.

6. Remove the airlocks, and reseal the jars with their lids. This ferment should store in a refrigerator for at least three months.

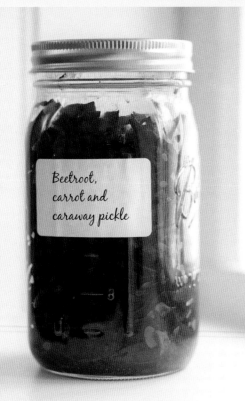

Beetroot, carrot and caraway pickle

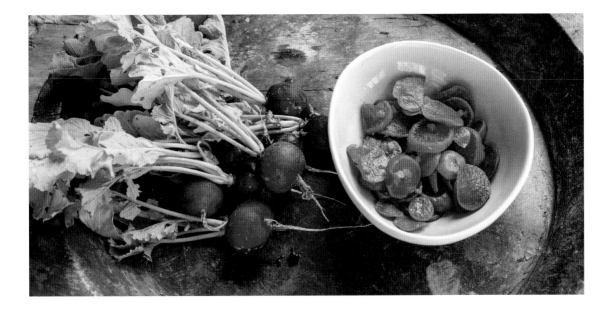

RADISH, TURMERIC AND CORIANDER PICKLE

Turmeric is one of my favourite spices. Its earthy bitterness pairs well with the pepperiness of the radish and the citrus tang of the coriander seed. Turmeric contains a potent polyphenol called curcumin which studies show is valuable in the fight against Crohn's disease, cancer, liver cirrhosis, lung disease, diabetes and Alzheimer's. When turmeric is fermented it actually makes more curcumin available for our bodies to absorb and increases the antioxidant activity. Fermentation really is alchemy.

Ingredients

700g/1lb 8oz radish
1 heaped tbsp unrefined sea salt
2 garlic cloves
1 tsp ground turmeric (or grow or buy fresh
    turmeric if you can get it and chop finely)
1 tsp crushed coriander seeds
2cm/1in piece of ginger, finely chopped

Method

1. Thinly slice the radish using a sharp knife.

2. Rub in the unrefined sea salt until you see the surface of the radish slices glistening with moisture.

3. Chop and crush the garlic. Stir all the ingredients, including the ground or fresh turmeric, into the salty radish mix.

4. Pack the ingredients tightly into a large mason jar. Weigh down the ingredients with a glass weight to ensure they are submerged under the brine.

5. Leave to ferment at room temperature for 5–7 days or until it reaches your preferred degree of sourness.

6. Remove the airlock, and reseal the jar with a lid. This ferment should store in a refrigerator for at least three months.

Late-summer & autumn recipes

FIERY FERMENT WITH CHILLI, PERILLA AND OREGANO

For those people like me and my family who add chilli sauce to virtually every meal, this one is for you. Each autumn we have a glut of chillies and this fermented sauce offers a perfect way to preserve and use our bounty through the winter months. The fermentation process gives the sauce a wonderful, almost smoky, tangy flavour. You can use your chillies from the 'Ferment planters' project on page 149 for the recipe.

Ingredients

500g/1lb 2oz chillies (approximately 25 chillies, or however many you have from your plants)
Unrefined sea salt (see method for guidance on exact salt quantities)
Large handful of chopped perilla leaves
Large handful of chopped oregano leaves

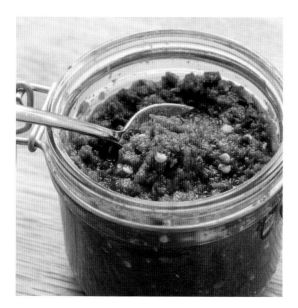

Method

1. Roughly chop the chillies, including the seed for an extra spicy kick.

2. Weigh your chillies and calculate how much unrefined sea salt you need. This should be 2 per cent of the weight of the chillies. For example, if your chillies weigh 500g/1lb 2oz you will need 1 tablespoon of sea salt.

3. Wearing gloves, rub in the salt until you can see the chillies glistening with the water that quickly starts to seep from the fruits. It's important to wear gloves for this step, otherwise your hands will really feel the burn of the chillies.

4. Mix in your chopped herbs.

5. Pack tightly into a one or two jars and seal each with an airlock (see page 165).

6. Leave for approximately two weeks at room temperature, although you can leave this ferment for longer if you prefer a really sour taste.

7. Blend the chilli and herb mix roughly and return it to the jar. You can also add a few chopped garlic cloves or some chopped ginger at this point, to add extra flavour to the sauce.

8. Store in the refrigerator and it should keep for a few months (although ours never lasts that long). If you do get any white mould forming at the top of the ferment, simply remove it.

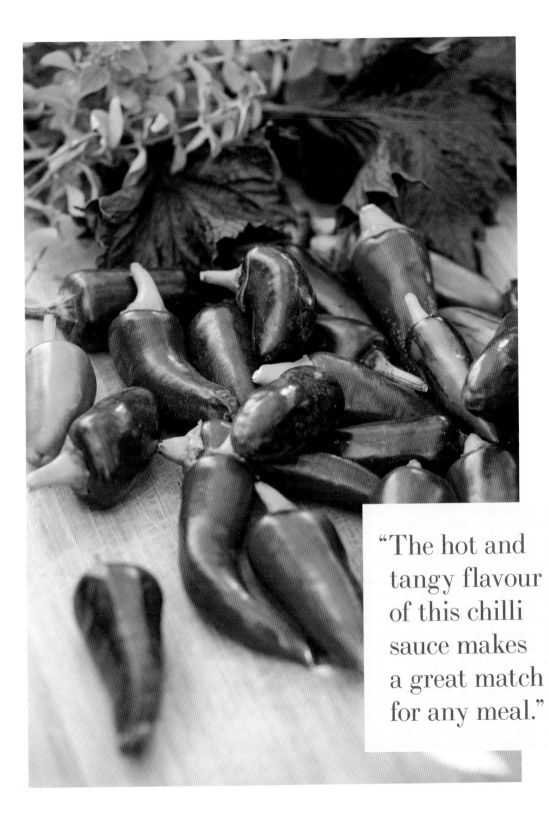

"The hot and tangy flavour of this chilli sauce makes a great match for any meal."

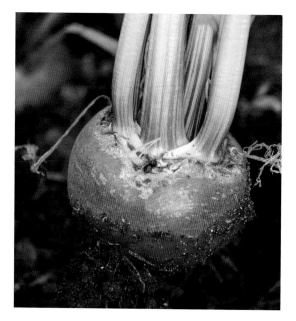

BEETROOT, APPLE AND ROSEMARY PICKLE

This ferment recipe has a lovely blend of sweetness from the apple and earthiness from the beetroot and rosemary. It's a great recipe for late summer when the apples are ready to harvest and you have more beetroot than you know what to do with. I've found this is a wonderful pickle to include in more or less any type of sandwich or with cheese.

Ingredients

900g/1lb 15oz beetroot
200g/7oz apple
1½ tbsp unrefined sea salt
Large handful of fresh rosemary

Method

1. Slice the beetroot and apple to the desired thickness. I slice mine thinly with a mandolin.

2. Rub in the sea salt thoroughly until the mixture is glistening with moisture from the beetroot and apple slices.

3. Chop the rosemary roughly and add it to the mix.

4. Pack the ingredients tightly into wide-mouthed mason jars. Weigh the ingredients down with glass weights to ensure they stay submerged under the salty brine.

5. Seal each jar with an airlock (see page 165) and leave to ferment at room temperature for 5–7 days or until you are happy with the sourness of the flavour.

6. Remove the airlocks and reseal the jars with their lids. This ferment should store in the refrigerator for a few months at least.

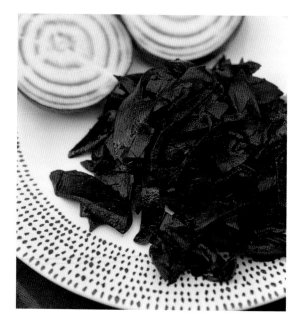

SPICY SEAKALE WITH FENNEL AND CHIVES

The Florence fennel in this recipe provides a crunchy texture and a pleasingly mild liquorice flavour. It is best to sow fennel from early to midsummer for an autumn harvest, or it can have a tendency to bolt. This ferment is a great spicy twist on traditional kimchi, using seakale (see page 166), together with chives and Florence fennel fresh from the garden.

Ingredients

750g/1lb 10oz seakale
500g/1lb 2oz Florence fennel
Large handful of chives
2 heaped tbsp unrefined sea salt
3 cloves of garlic
1 tbsp gochugaru (Korean red pepper
   flakes) or chilli flakes

Method

1. Finely chop the seakale, Florence fennel and the chives.

2. Rub in the unrefined sea salt. The seakale has a really high moisture content so you'll find it releases masses of liquid when you add the salt.

3. Crush and chop the garlic. Stir the garlic and gochugaru (or chilli flakes) into the mixture.

4. Pack tightly into mason jars. Submerge the vegetables under the brine using glass weights, then seal each with an airlock (see page 165).

5. Leave to ferment at room temperature for 5–7 days or until it reaches the sourness you like. Remove the airlocks and reseal with lids. This ferment should store in the refrigerator for at least a few months.

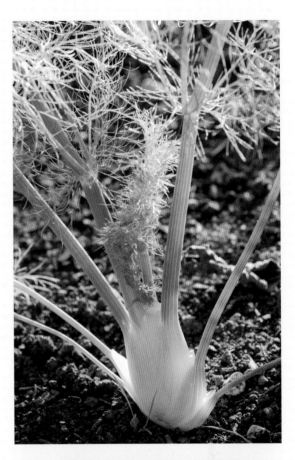

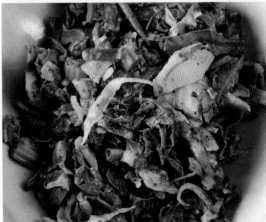

Winter recipes

TRADITIONAL SAUERKRAUT

Crunchy cabbage, sweet carrot, a hint of bitter lemony aniseed from dill – this classic pickle is resoundingly popular with good reason. It can be made using traditional white cabbage, or try red cabbage instead for a colourful alternative. Use your home-grown ingredients from the Ferment Planters project on page 148 to make this recipe.

Ingredients

800g–1kg/1lb 12oz–2lb 3oz cabbage
2–3 carrots
1½ tbsp unrefined sea salt
Handful of chopped dill
1 tbsp caraway seeds (these are optional but make a delicious addition)

Method

1. Slice the cabbage and carrots to the desired thickness – I use a mandolin for thin slices.

2. Rub the sea salt into the cabbage and carrots thoroughly. The proportion of salt should be 2 per cent of the total weight of the cabbages and carrots, so check and adapt the salt levels as necessary.

3. Stir in the chopped dill.

4. Pack all the ingredients tightly into mason jars using a tamper. Place glass weights on top to help submerge the sauerkraut under the brine.

5. Seal with airlocks (see page 165) and leave for 5–7 days at room temperature, or longer if you want a sourer taste. Remove the airlocks, seal the jars with their lids and store in the refrigerator. The sauerkraut will keep for three months or more.

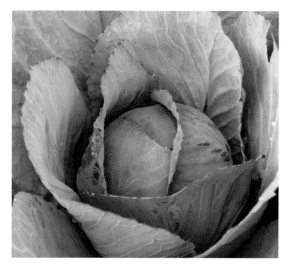

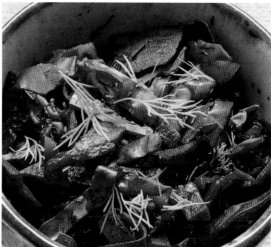

CELERIAC, APPLE, LEMON AND MUSTARD SEED KRAUT

The crunchy, mild celery flavour of celeriac makes it an excellent vegetable to ferment. Combined with the sweetness of the apple and bitterness of mustard seeds, this is my favourite winter ferment. It's great in sandwiches and I also love it with avocado on toast.

Ingredients

900g/1lb 15oz celeriac
200g/7oz apples
1 tbsp black mustard seeds
1 lemon
1½ tbsp unrefined sea salt

Method

1. Finely slice the celeriac and apples with a mandolin and chop into strips.

2. Rub the unrefined sea salt into the ingredients thoroughly until they start to release moisture.

3. Stir in the mustard seeds and the zest and juice of the lemon.

4. Pack the ingredients tightly into wide-mouthed mason jars, pressing them down firmly with a tamper.

5. Weigh the mixture down with glass weights to ensure it remains submerged under the brine. Seal the jars with airlocks (see p165).

6. Leave the ingredients to ferment for 5–7 days at room temperature or until it has developed the degree of pickliness you prefer.

7. Remove the airlocks and reseal the jars with their lids. This ferment should store in a refrigerator for a minimum of three months.

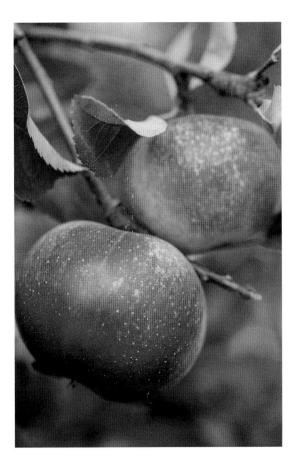

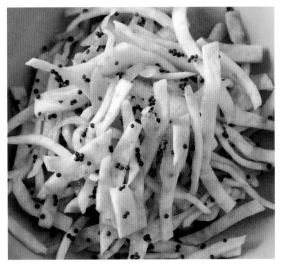

References

INTRODUCTION

Johnson, A. J., et al. 2019. 'Daily sampling reveals personalized diet-microbiome associations in humans.' *Cell Host & Microbe, 25(6), 789–802.*

Le Roy, C., et al. 2019. 'Red wine consumption associated with increased gut microbiota α-diversity in 3 independent cohorts.' *Gastroenterology*, S0016-5085(19), 41244-4.

McDonald D., et al. 2018. 'American Gut: an open platform for citizen science microbiome research.' mSystems3: e00031-18.

THE SCIENCE EXPLAINED

Barański, M., et al. 2014. 'Higher antioxidant and lower cadmium concentrations and lower incidence of pesticide residues in organically grown crops: a systematic literature review.' *British Journal of Nutrition*, 112(05), 794–811.

Baudry J, Assmann KE, Touvier M, et al. 2018. 'Association of frequency of organic food consumption with cancer risk: findings from the NutriNet-Santé prospective cohort study.' *JAMA Internal Medicine*, 178(12): 1597–1606.

Berg, G., & Raaijmakers, J. M. 2018. 'Saving seed microbiomes.' *The ISME Journal*, 12(5), 1167–1170.

Berni, R., et al. 2018. 'Agrobiotechnology goes wild: ancient local varieties as sources of bioactives.' *International Journal of Molecular Sciences*, 19(8), 2248.

Berry Ottaway, P. (2010). 'Stability of vitamins during food processing and storage.' *Chemical Deterioration and Physical Instability of Food and Beverages*, 539–560.

Blaser M.J. 2016. 'Antibiotic use and its consequences for the normal microbiome.' *Science, 352:544-5.*

Blum, W., et al. 2019. 'Does soil contribute to the human gut microbiome?' *Microorganisms, 7*(9), 287.

Bonder MJ, Tigchelaar EF, Cai X, et al. 2016. 'The influence of a short-term gluten-free diet on the human gut microbiome.' *Genome Med,* Apr 21; 8(1):45.

Cevallos-Casals, B. A., & Cisneros-Zevallos, L. 2010. 'Impact of germination on phenolic content and antioxidant activity of 13 edible seed species.' *Food Chemistry*, 119(4), 1485–1490.

Cheynier, V. 2005. 'Polyphenols in foods are more complex than often thought.' *American Journal of Clinical Nutrition, 81, 223S–229S.*

Clemente, J. C., et al. 2012. 'The impact of the gut microbiota on human health: an integrative view.' *Cell*, 148(6), 1258–1270.

Compant, S., et al. 2019. 'A review on the plant microbiome: Ecology, functions and emerging trends in microbial application.' *Journal of Advanced Research*, 19, 29-37.

D'Archivio, M., Filesi, C., Varì, R., Scazzocchio, B., & Masella, R. 2010. 'Bioavailability of the polyphenols: status and controversies.'

International Journal of Molecular Sciences, 11(4), 1321–1342.

Drewnowski, A., & Gomez-Carneros, C. 2000. 'Bitter taste, phytonutrients, and the consumer: a review.' *The American Journal of Clinical Nutrition*, 72(6), 1424–1435.

Ezekiel, R., Singh, N., Sharma, S., & Kaur, A. 2013. 'Beneficial phytochemicals in potato — a review.' *Food Research International*, 50(2), 487–496.

Fei, M. L., Tong, L., Wei, L., & De Yang, L. 2015. 'Changes in antioxidant capacity, levels of soluble sugar, total polyphenol, organosulfur compound and constituents in garlic clove during storage.' *Industrial Crops and Products*, 69, 137–142.

Food and Agriculture Organization of the United Nations (FAO). 2018. 'Biodiversity for sustainable agriculture: fao's work on biodiversity for food and agriculture.', *FAO.*

Food and Agriculture Organization of the United Nations (FAO). 2014. 'Promotion of underutilized indigenous food resources for food security and nutrition in Asia and the Pacific.', FAO.

Gibson, G. R., et al. 2017. 'Expert consensus document: The International Scientific Association for Probiotics and Prebiotics consensus statement on the definition and scope of prebiotics.' *Nature Reviews Gastroenterology & Hepatology.*

Gibson, P.R. 2017. 'The evidence base for efficacy of the low FODMAP diet in irritable bowel syndrome?' *Journal of Gastroenterology Hepatology, 32(Suppl 1):32-5.*

Giovanelli, G., & Buratti, S. 2009. 'Comparison of polyphenolic composition and antioxidant activity of wild Italian blueberries and some cultivated varieties.' *Food Chemistry*, 112(4), 903–908.

Goodrich, J. K., et al. 2014. 'Human genetics shape the gut microbiome.' *Cell*, 159(4), 789–799.

Grönroos, M., Parajuli, A., et al. 2018. 'Short-term direct contact with soil and plant materials leads to an immediate increase in diversity of skin microbiota.' *MicrobiologyOpen*, e00645.

Guallar, E., et al. 2013. 'Enough is enough: stop wasting money on vitamin and mineral supplements.' *Annals of Internal Medicine*, 159(12), 850–851.

Harbourne, N., et al. 2013. 'Stability of phytochemicals as sources of anti-inflammatory nutraceuticals in beverages — A review.' *Food Research International*, 50(2), 480–486.

Hehemann, J.-H., et al. 2010. 'Transfer of carbohydrate-active enzymes from marine bacteria to Japanese gut microbiota.' *Nature*, 464(7290), 908–912.

Hill, C., et al. 2014. 'The International Scientific Association for Probiotics and Prebiotics consensus statement on the scope and appropriate use of the term probiotic.' *Nature Reviews Gastroenterology & Hepatology*, 11(8), 506–514.

Hooper, B., Spiro, A., & Stanner, S. 2015. '30 g of fibre a day: An achievable recommendation?' *Nutrition Bulletin*, 40(2), 118–129.

Hur, S. J., et al. 2014. 'Effect of fermentation on the antioxidant activity in plant-based foods.' *Food Chemistry*, 160, 346–356.

Jackson A., M., et al. 2018. 'Gut microbiota

associations with common diseases and prescription medications in a population-based cohort.' *Nature Communications*, 9, Article number: 2655.

Jacobsen, C. S., & Hjelmsø, M. H. 2014. 'Agricultural soils, pesticides and microbial diversity.' *Current Opinion in Biotechnology*, 27, 15–20.

Jazić, M., et al. 2018. 'Polyphenolic composition, antioxidant and antiproliferative effects of wild and cultivated blackberries.' *International Journal of Food Science & Technology*, 54(1), 194-201.

Liu, H., et al. 2018. 'Butyrate: a double-edged sword for health?' *Advances in Nutrition*, 9(1), 21–29.

Livingston, D. P., Hincha, D. K., & Heyer, A. G. 2009. 'Fructan and its relationship to abiotic stress tolerance in plants.' *Cellular and Molecular Life Sciences*, 66(13), 2007–2023.

Maier, L., et al. 2018. 'Extensive impact of non-antibiotic drugs on human gut bacteria.' *Nature,* 555(7698), 623–628.

Mansoorian, B., et al. 2019. 'Impact of fermentable fibres on the colonic microbiota metabolism of dietary polyphenols rutin and quercetin.' *International Journal of Environmental Research and Public Health*, 16(2), 292.

Perez-Jimenez J., et al. 2010. 'Identification of the 100 richest dietary sources of polyphenols.' *European Journal Clinical Nutrition; 64(S3): S112-S120.*

Premier, R. 2002. 'Phytochemical composition: A paradigm shift for food-health considerations.' *Asia Pacific Journal of Clinical Nutrition*, 11(s6), S197–S201.

Reijnders D., et al. 2016. 'Effects of gut microbiota manipulation by antibiotics on host metabolism in obese humans.' *Cell Metabolism*, 24:63-74.

Roberfroid, M.B. 2007. 'Inulin-type fructans: functional food ingredients.' *The Journal of Nutrition*, 137 (11), 2493–2502.

Rossi, M., et al. 2005 'Fermentation of fructooligosaccharides and inulin by bifidobacteria: a comparative study of pure and fecal cultures.' *Applied and Environmental Microbiology*, 71(10), 6150–6158.

Sender, R., Fuchs, S., & Milo, R. 2016. 'Revised estimates for the number of human and bacteria cells in the body.' *PLOS Biology,* 14(8).

Smith-Spangler, C., 2012. 'Are organic foods safer or healthier than conventional alternatives?' *Annals of Internal Medicine*, 157(5), 348.

Smith-Spangler, C., et al. 2012. 'Are organic foods safer or healthier than conventional alternatives?' *Annals of Internal Medicine*, 157(5), 348.

Sonnenburg E. D., et al. 2016. 'Diet-induced extinctions in the gut microbiota compound over generations.' *Nature* 529(7585), 212.

Thakur, A. and Sharma, R. 2018. 'Health promoting phytochemicals in vegetables: A mini review.' *International Journal Food Fermented Technology 8(2): 107-117.*

Tomova, A., et al. 2019. 'The effects of vegetarian and vegan diets on gut microbiota.' *Frontiers in Nutrition*, 6: 47.

Trevors, J. T. 2009. 'One gram of soil: a

microbial biochemical gene library.' *Antonie van Leeuwenhoek*, 97(2), 99–106.

Valdes, A. M., Walter, J., Segal, E., & Spector, T. D. 2018. 'Role of the gut microbiota in nutrition and health.' *British Medical Journal*, k2179.

Vallejo, F., Tomás-Barberán, F., & García-Viguera, C. 2003. 'Health-promoting compounds in broccoli as influenced by refrigerated transport and retail sale period.' *Journal of Agricultural and Food Chemistry*, 51(10), 3029–3034.

Van Bruggen, et al. 2018. 'Environmental and health effects of the herbicide glyphosate.' *Science of The Total Environment*, 616-617, 255–268.

Verkerk, R., et al. 2008. 'Glucosinolates in Brassica vegetables: The influence of the food supply chain on intake, bioavailability and human health.' *Molecular Nutrition & Food Research*, 53(S2), S219–S219.

Wassermann, et al. 2019. 'An apple a day: which bacteria do we eat with organic and conventional apples?' *Frontiers in Microbiology*, 10.

Wu, G. D., Compher, et al. 2014. 'Comparative metabolomics in vegans and omnivores reveal constraints on diet-dependent gut microbiota metabolite production.' *Gut*, 65(1), 63–72.

Zinöcker, M., & Lindseth, I. 2018. 'The Western Diet–microbiome-host interaction and its role in metabolic disease.' *Nutrients*, 10(3), 365.

VEGETABLES & FRUIT IN FOCUS

The onion family

Bernaert, N. 2013. 'Bioactive compounds in leek (*Allium ampeloprasum* var. *porrum*): Analysis as a function of the genetic diversity, harvest time and processing techniques'. Ghent, Belgium: Ghent University. Faculty of Bioscience Engineering.

Bloem, E., Haneklaus, S., & Schnug, E. 2010. 'influence of fertilizer practices on s-containing metabolites in garlic (*Allium sativum* L.) under field conditions.' *Journal of Agricultural and Food Chemistry*, 58(19), 10690–10696.

Griffiths, G. et al. 2002. 'Onions? A global benefit to health.' *Phytotherapy Research*, 16(7), 603–615.

Hedges, L & Lister, Carolyn. 2007. 'The nutritional attributes of Allium species.' *New Zealand Institute for Crop & Food Research Limited*.

Jones, M.G. et al. 2007. 'The biochemical and physiological genesis of alliin in garlic.' *Medicinal Aromatic Plant Science and Biotechnology*, 1. 21-24.

Leskovar, D. I., Crosby, K., & Jifon, J. L. 2009. 'Impact of agronomic practices on phytochemicals and quality of vegetable crops.' *Acta Horticulturae*, (841), 317–322.

Martins, N., et al. 2016. 'Chemical composition and bioactive compounds of garlic (*Allium sativum* L.) as affected by pre- and post-harvest conditions: A review.' *Food Chemistry*, 211, 41–50.

Nencini, C. et al. 2007. 'Evaluation of antioxidative properties of Allium species growing wild in Italy.' *Phytotherapy Research*, 21(9), 874–878.

Pérez-Gregorio, et al. 2010. 'Identification and quantification of flavonoids in traditional cultivars of red and white onions at harvest.' *Journal of Food Composition and Analysis*, 23(6), 592–598.

Perner, H., et al. 2008. 'Effect of nitrogen species supply and mycorrhizal colonization on organosulfur and phenolic compounds in onions.' *Journal of Agricultural and Food Chemistry*, 56(10), 3538–3545.

Pöhnl, T., Schweiggert, R. M., & Carle, R. 2018. 'Impact of cultivation method and cultivar selection on soluble carbohydrates and pungent principles in onions (*Allium cepa* L.).' *Journal of Agricultural and Food Chemistry*, 66(48), 12827-12835

Prati, P., et al. 2014. 'Evaluation of allicin stability in processed garlic of different cultivars.' *Food Science and Technology*, 34(3), 623–628.

Rodrigues, A. S., et al. 2017. 'Onions: A source of flavonoids – from biosynthesis to human health.' *Ebook (PDF) ISBN: 978-953-51-4697-1*

Rodrigues, A. S., et al 2011. 'Effect of meteorological conditions on antioxidant flavonoids in Portuguese cultivars of white and red onions.' *Food Chemistry*, 124(1), 303–308.

Thompson, M. D., & Thompson, H. J. 2010. 'Botanical diversity in vegetable and fruit intake.' *Bioactive Foods in Promoting Health*, 1–17.

The carrot family

Alasalvar, C., et al. 2001. 'Comparison of volatiles, phenolics, sugars, antioxidant vitamins, and sensory quality of different colored carrot varieties.' *Journal of Agricultural and Food Chemistry*, 49(3), 1410–1416.

Grassmann, J., et al. 2007. 'Evaluation of different coloured carrot cultivars on antioxidative capacity based on their carotenoid and phenolic contents.' *International Journal of Food Sciences and Nutrition*, 58(8), 603–611.

Kidmose, U., et al 2006. 'Effects of genotype, root size, storage, and processing on bioactive compounds in organically grown carrots.' *Journal of Food Science*, 69(9), S388–S394.

Montilla, E. C., et al. 2011. 'Anthocyanin composition of black carrot cultivars Antonina, Beta Sweet, Deep Purple, and Purple Haze.' *Journal of Agricultural and Food Chemistry*, 59(7), 3385–3390.

Phan, C.T., and Hsu, H. 1973. 'Physical and chemical changes occurring in the carrot root during growth.' *Canadian Journal of Plant Science*, 53(3), 629–634.

Sharma, K. D., Karki, S., Thakur, N. S., & Attri, S. 2011. 'Chemical composition, functional properties and processing of carrot—a review.' *Journal of Food Science and Technology*, 49(1), 22–32.

Singh, D. P., Beloy, J., McInerney, J. K., & Day, L. 2012. 'Impact of boron, calcium and genetic factors on vitamin C, carotenoids, phenolic acids, anthocyanins and antioxidant capacity of carrots.' *Food Chemistry*, 132(3), 1161–1170.

Wruss, J., et al. 2015. 'Compositional characteristics of commercial beetroot products and beetroot juice prepared from seven beetroot varieties grown in Upper Austria.' *Journal of Food Composition and Analysis*, 42, 46–55.

Zhang, Donglin & Hamauzu, Yasunori. 2004. 'Phenolic compounds and their antioxidant properties in different tissues of carrots.' *Journal of Food Agriculture and Environment, 2(1).*

The beet family

Chaturvedi, N., et al. 2013. 'Comparative nutritional and phytochemical analysis of spinach cultivars: *B. alba* and *S. oleracea.*' *International Journal of Research in Pharmaceutical and Biomedical Sciences*, 4(2), 674-679

Clifford, T., et al. 2015. 'The potential benefits of red beetroot supplementation in health and disease.' *Nutrients*, 7(4), 2801–2822.

Howard, L. R., Pandjaitan, N., Morelock, T., & Gil, M. I. 2002. 'Antioxidant capacity and phenolic content of spinach as affected by genetics and growing season.' *Journal of Agricultural and Food Chemistry*, 50(21), 5891–5896.

Kugler, F., et al. 2004. 'Identification of betalains from petioles of differently colored Swiss chard (*Beta vulgaris* L. ssp. *cicla* [L.] Alef. cv. Bright Lights) by high-performance liquid chromatography–electrospray ionization mass spectrometry.' *Journal of Agricultural and Food Chemistry*, 52(10), 2975–2981.

Kujala, T. S., et al. 2000. 'Phenolics and betacyanins in red beetroot (*Beta vulgaris*) root: distribution and effect of cold storage on the content of total phenolics and three individual compounds.' *Journal of Agricultural and Food Chemistry,* 48(11), 5338–5342.

Lee, E. J., et al. 2014. 'Betalain and betaine composition of greenhouse- or field-produced beetroot (*Beta vulgaris* L.) and Inhibition of HepG2 cell proliferation.' *Journal of Agricultural and Food Chemistry*, 62(6), 1324–1331.

Lester, G. E., Makus, D. J., & Hodges, D. M. 2010. 'Relationship between fresh-packaged spinach leaves exposed to continuous light or dark and bioactive contents: effects of cultivar, leaf size, and storage duration.' *Journal of Agricultural and Food Chemistry*, 58(5), 2980–2987.

Murphy, M., et al. 2012. 'Whole beetroot consumption acutely improves running performance.' *Journal of the Academy of Nutrition and Dietetics, 112(4), 548–552.*

Nizioł-Łukaszewska, Z., & Gawęda, M. 2014. 'Changes in quality of selected red beet (Beta vulgaris L.) cultivars during the growing season.' *Folia Horticulturae*, 26(2), 139–146.

Pandjaitan, N., et al. 2005. 'Antioxidant capacity and phenolic content of spinach as affected by genetics and maturation.' *Journal of Agricultural and Food Chemistry*, 53(22), 8618–8623.

Pyo, Y.-H., et al. 2004. 'Antioxidant activity and phenolic compounds of Swiss chard (*Beta vulgaris* subspecies *cycla*) extracts.' *Food Chemistry*, 85(1), 19–26.

Rani E.P., Fernando, R.R.S. 2016. 'Effect of cooking on total antioxidant activity in selected vegetables.' *International Journal of Home Science, 2(2), 218-222.*

Roberts, J. L., & Moreau, R. 2016. 'Functional properties of spinach (*Spinacia oleracea* L.) phytochemicals and bioactives.' *Food & Function*, 7(8), 3337–3353.

Rouphael, Y., et al. 2018. 'Plant- and seaweed-based extracts increase yield but differentially modulate nutritional quality of greenhouse spinach through biostimulant action.' *Agronomy*, 8(7), 126.

Slatnar, A., et al. 2015. 'HPLC-msnidentification of betalain profile of different beetroot (*Beta vulgaris* L.ssp. *vulgaris*) parts and cultivars.' *Journal of Food Science*, 80(9), C1952–C1958.

Vinson, J. A., Hao, Y., Su, X., & Zubik, L. 1998. 'Phenol antioxidant quantity and quality in foods: vegetables.' *Journal of Agricultural and Food Chemistry*, 46(9), 3630–3634.

Wang, M., et al. 2017. 'Limited tyrosine utilization explains lower betalain contents in yellow than in red table beet genotypes.' *Journal of Agricultural and Food Chemistry*, 65(21), 4305–4313.

The asparagus family
Kulczyński B., et al. 2016. 'Antiradical capacity and polyphenol composition of asparagus spears varieties cultivated under different sunlight conditions.' *Acta Scientiarum Polonorum Technologia Alimentaria*, 15 (3), 267-279.

Maeda, Tomoo, et al. 2005. 'Antioxidation capacities of extracts from green, purple, and white asparagus spears related to polyphenol concentration.' *HortScience, 40(5)*.

Makris, D. P., & Rossiter, J. T. 2001. 'Domestic processing of onion bulbs and asparagus spears: Effect on flavonol content and antioxidant status.' *Journal of Agricultural and Food Chemistry, 49(7), 3216–3222.*

Stoffyn, O. M., Tsao, R., Liu, R., & Wolyn, D. J. 2012. 'The effects of environment and storage on rutin concentration in two asparagus cultivars grown in southern Ontario.' *Canadian Journal of Plant Science*, 92(5), 901–912.

The sunflower family
Ahmed, W., & Rashid, S. 2017. 'Functional and therapeutic potential of inulin: A comprehensive review.' *Critical Reviews in Food Science and Nutrition*, 1–13.

Bach, V., Clausen, M. R., & Edelenbos, M. 2015. 'Production of Jerusalem artichoke and impact on inulin and phenolic compounds.' *Processing and Impact on Active Components in Food*, 97–102.

Bach, V., et al. 2013. 'The effect of culinary preparation on carbohydrate composition, texture and sensory quality of Jerusalem artichoke tubers (*Helianthus tuberosus* L.).' *LWT - Food Science and Technology*, 54(1), 165–170.

Boo, H.-O., et al. 2011. 'Positive effects of temperature and growth conditions on enzymatic and antioxidant status in lettuce plants.' *Plant Science*, 181(4), 479–484.

Ceccarelli, N., et al. 2010. 'Globe artichoke as a functional food.' *Mediterranean Journal of Nutrition and Metabolism*, 3(3), 197–201.

Costabile, A., et al. 2010. 'A double-blind, placebo-controlled, cross-over study to establish the bifidogenic effect of a very-long-chain inulin extracted from globe artichoke (*Cynara scolymus*) in healthy human subjects.' *British Journal of Nutrition*, 104(07), 1007–1017.

Fratianni, F., et al. 2007. 'Polyphenolic composition in different parts of some cultivars of globe artichoke (*Cynara cardunculus* L. *var. scolymus* (L.) Fiori).' *Food Chemistry*, 104(3), 1282–1286.

Lattanzio, V., Kroon, P. A., Linsalata, V., & Cardinali, A. 2009. 'Globe artichoke: A functional food and source of nutraceutical ingredients.' *Journal of Functional Foods, 1(2), 131–144.*

Llorach, R., et al. 2008. 'Characterisation of polyphenols and antioxidant properties of five lettuce varieties and escarole.' *Food Chemistry*, 108(3), 1028–1038.

Martínez-Esplá, A., et al. 2017. 'Preharvest application of oxalic acid improves quality and phytochemical content of artichoke at harvest and during storage.' *Food Chemistry*, 230, 343–349.

Milala, J. et al. 2009. 'Composition and properties of chicory extracts rich in fructans and polyphenols.' *Polish Journal of Food and Nutritional Sciences*, 59(1), 35-43

Negro, D., et al. 2012. 'Polyphenol compounds in artichoke plant tissues and varieties.' *Journal of Food Science*, 77(2), C244–C252.

Pandino, G., et al. 2013. 'Choice of time of harvest influences the polyphenol profile of globe artichoke.' *Journal of Functional Foods*, 5(4), 1822–1828.

Puangbut; et al. 2012. 'Influence of planting date and temperature on inulin content in Jerusalem artichoke'. *Australian Journal of Crop Science*: 1159–1165.

Renna, M., Gonnella, M., Giannino, D., & Santamaria, P. 2013. 'Quality evaluation of cook-chilled chicory stems by conventional and sous-vide cooking methods.' *Journal of the Science of Food and Agriculture, 94(4), 656–665.*

Romani, A., et al. 2002. 'Polyphenols in greenhouse and open-air-grown lettuce.' *Food Chemistry*, 79(3), 337–342.

Rubel, I. A., et al. 2014. 'In vitro prebiotic activity of inulin-rich carbohydrates extracted from Jerusalem artichoke tubers at different storage times by *Lactobacillus paracasei*'. *Food Research International*, 62, 59–65.

Sinkovic, L. et al. 2014. 'Influence of cultivar and storage of chicory (*Cichorium intybus* L.) plants on polyphenol composition and antioxidative potential.' *Czech Journal of Food Science, Vol. 32, 2014, No. 1: 10–15.*

Van Loo, J., et al. 1995. 'On the presence of inulin and oligofructose as natural ingredients in the western diet.' *Critical Reviews in Food Science and Nutrition*, 35(6), 525–552.

Wilson, R. G., Smith, J. A., & Yonts, C. D. 2004. 'Chicory root yield and carbohydrate composition is influenced by cultivar selection, planting, and harvest date.' *Crop Science*, 44(3), 748.

Zhao, X., Carey, E. E., Young, J. E., Wang, W., & Iwamoto, T. 2007. 'Influences of organic fertilization, high tunnel environment, and postharvest storage on phenolic compounds in lettuce.' *HortScience horts*, 42(1), 71-76.

Zubr, J., Pedersen, H.S. 1993. 'Characteristics of growth and development of different Jerusalem artichoke cultivars', in *Studies in Plant Science*, Elsevier.

The cabbage family
Ahmed, F. A., & Ali, R. F. M. 2013. 'Bioactive compounds and antioxidant activity of fresh and processed white cauliflower.' *BioMed Research International*, 2013, 1–9.

Björkman, M., et al. 2011. 'Phytochemicals of *Brassicaceae* in plant protection and human health – Influences of climate, environment and agronomic practice.' *Phytochemistry*, 72(7), 538–556.

Cartea, M. E., & Velasco, P. 2007. 'Glucosinolates in Brassica foods: bioavailability in food and significance for human health.' *Phytochemistry Reviews*, 7(2), 213–229.

Charron, C. S., Saxton, A. M., & Sams, C. E. 2005. 'Relationship of climate and genotype to seasonal variation in the glucosinolate-myrosinase system. I. Glucosinolate content in ten cultivars of *Brassica oleracea* grown in fall and spring seasons.' *Journal of the Science of Food and Agriculture*, 85(4), 671–681.

Ciska, Ewa & Karamać, Magdalena & Kosinska, Agnieszka. 2005. 'Antioxidant activity of extracts of white cabbage and sauerkraut.' *Polish Journal of Food and Nutrition Sciences*, 55(4), 367-373.

Doorn, J.E. van. 1999. 'Development of vegetables with improved consumer quality: a case study in Brussels sprouts.' Agricultural University, W.M.F. Jongen, L.H.W. van der Plas.

Fahey, J. W., Zhang, Y., & Talalay, P. 1997. 'Broccoli sprouts: An exceptionally rich source of inducers of enzymes that protect against chemical carcinogens.' *Proceedings of the National Academy of Sciences*, 94(19).

Fortier, E., et al. 2010. 'Influence of irrigation and nitrogen fertilization on broccoli polyphenolics concentration.' *Acta Horticulturae*, (856), 55–62.

Francisco, M., et al. 2016. 'Nutritional and phytochemical value of Brassica crops from the agri-food perspective.' *Annals of Applied Biology*, 170(2), 273–285.

Gols, R., et al, 2008. 'Performance of generalist and specialist herbivores and their endoparasitoids differs on cultivated and wild Brassica populations.' *Journal of Chemical Ecology*, 34, 132–143.

Gratacós-Cubarsí, M., et al. 2010. 'Simultaneous evaluation of intact glucosinolates and phenolic compounds by UPLC-DAD-MS/MS in *Brassica oleracea* L. var. *botrytis*.' *Food Chemistry*, 121(1), 257–263.

Jahangir, M., et al. 2009. 'Healthy and unhealthy plants: The effect of stress on the metabolism of Brassicaceae.' *Environmental and Experimental Botany*, 67(1), 23–33.

Ju-Sung, I., et al. 2010. 'Sulforaphane and total phenolics contents and antioxidant activity of radish according to genotype and cultivation location with different altitudes.' *Horticultural Science and Technology*, 28(3), 335-342.

Kałużewicz A., et al. 2017. 'The effects of plant density and irrigation on phenolic content in cauliflower.' *Horticultural Science (Prague)*, 44, 178–185.

Kurilich, A. C., et al. 1999. 'Carotene, tocopherol, and ascorbate contents in subspecies of *Brassica oleracea*.' *Journal of Agricultural and Food Chemistry*, 47(4), 1576–1581.

Kusznierewicz, B., et al. 2008. 'Partial characterization of white cabbages from different regions by glucosinolates, bioactive compounds, total antioxidant activities and proteins.' *LWT - Food Science and Technology*, 41(1), 1–9.

Li, H., et al. 2012. 'Highly pigmented vegetables: Anthocyanin compositions and their role in antioxidant activities.' *Food Research International*, 46(1), 250–259.

Lola-Luz, T., Hennequart, F., & Gaffney, M. 2014. 'Effect on yield, total phenolic, total flavonoid and total isothiocyanate content of two broccoli cultivars (*Brassica oleracea* var *italica*) following the application of a commercial brown seaweed extract (*Ascophyllum nodosum*).' *Agricultural and Food Science*, 23(1), 28-37.

Nilsson, J., et al. 2006. 'Variation in the content of glucosinolates, hydroxycinnamic acids, carotenoids, total antioxidant capacity and low-molecular-weight carbohydrates in Brassica vegetables.' *Journal of the Science of Food and Agriculture*, 86(4), 528–538.

Olsen, H., et al. 2012. 'Antiproliferative effects of fresh and thermal processed green and red cultivars of curly kale.' *Journal of Agricultural and Food Chemistry*, 60(30), 7375–7383.

Podse,dek, A., Sosnowska, D., Redzynia, M., & Anders, B. 2006. 'Antioxidant capacity and content of *Brassica oleracea* dietary antioxidants.' *International Journal of Food Science and Technology*, 41(s1), 49–58.

Rungapamestry, V., Duncan, A. J., Fuller, Z., & Ratcliffe, B. 2006. 'Changes in glucosinolate concentrations, myrosinase activity, and production of metabolites of glucosinolates in cabbage (*Brassica oleracea* var.*capitata*) cooked for different durations.' *Journal of Agricultural and Food Chemistry*, 54(20), 7628–7634.

Šamec, D., Urlić, B., & Salopek-Sondi, B. 2018. ‹Kale as a superfood: Review of the scientific evidence behind the statement.' *Critical Reviews in Food Science and Nutrition*, 1–12.

Sasaki, K., Neyazaki, M., Shindo, K., Ogawa, T., & Momose, M. 2012. 'Quantitative profiling of glucosinolates by LC–MS analysis reveals several cultivars of cabbage and kale as promising sources of sulforaphane.' *Journal of Chromatography B*, 903, 171–176.

Schonhof, I., et al. 2007. 'Sulfur and nitrogen supply influence growth, product appearance, and glucosinolate concentration of broccoli.' *Journal of Plant Nutrition and Soil Science*, 170(1), 65–72.

Shin, T., Ahn, M., Kim, G. O., & Park, S. U. 2015. 'Biological activity of various radish species.' *Oriental Pharmacy and Experimental Medicine*, 15(2), 105–111.

Singh, J., et al. 2006. 'Antioxidant phytochemicals in cabbage (*Brassica oleracea* L. var. *capitata*).' *Scientia Horticulturae*, 108(3), 233–237.

Singh, J., Upadhyay, A. K., Prasad, K., Bahadur, A., & Rai, M. 2007. 'Variability of carotenes, vitamin C, E and phenolics in Brassica vegetables.' *Journal of Food Composition and Analysis*, 20(2), 106–112.

Vallejo, F., Tomás-Barberán, F., & García-Viguera, C. 2003. 'Health-promoting compounds in broccoli as influenced by refrigerated transport and retail sale period.' *Journal of Agricultural and Food Chemistry*, 51(10), 3029–3034.

Verkerk, R., et al. 2008. 'Glucosinolates in Brassica vegetables: The influence of the food supply chain on intake, bioavailability and human health.' *Molecular Nutrition & Food Research*, 53(S2), S219–S219.

Verkerk, R., Tebbenhoff, S., & Dekker, M. 2010. 'Variation and distribution of glucosinolates in 42 varieties of *Brassica oleracea* vegetable crops.' *Acta Horticulturae*, (856), 63–70.

Volden, J., Borge, G. I. A., Hansen, M., Wicklund, T., & Bengtsson, G. B. 2009. 'Processing (blanching, boiling, steaming) effects on the content of glucosinolates and antioxidant-related parameters in cauliflower.' *LWT - Food Science and Technology*, 42(1), 63–73.

Walsh, R. P., Bartlett, H., & Eperjesi, F. 2015. 'Variation in carotenoid content of kale and other vegetables: a review of pre- and post-harvest effects.' *Journal of Agricultural and Food Chemistry*, 63(44), 9677–9682.

Wang, J., Zhao, Z., Sheng, X., Yu, H., & Gu, H. 2015. 'Influence of leaf-cover on visual quality and health-promoting phytochemicals in loose-curd cauliflower florets.' *LWT - Food Science and Technology*, 61(1), 177–183.

Yan-Wu, L. et al. 2014. 'Effects of light quality on total phenolic contents and antioxidant activity in radish sprouts.' *Acta Horticulturae Sinica*, 2014-03.

Yuan, G., Sun, B., Yuan, J., & Wang, Q. 2009. 'Effects of different cooking methods on health-promoting compounds of broccoli.' *Journal of Zhejiang University*, 10(8), 580–588.

The squash family
Antonia Murcia, M., Jiménez, A. M., & Martínez-Tomé, M. 2009. 'Vegetables antioxidant losses during industrial processing and refrigerated storage.' *Food Research International*, 42(8), 1046–1052.

Baljeet, S.Y., Roshanlal, Y. and Ritika, B.Y. 2016. 'Effect of cooking methods and extraction solvents on the antioxidant activity of summer squash vegetable extracts.' *International Food Research Journal*, 23(4), 1531-1540.

Del Río-Celestino, M., et al. 2012. 'Quantification of carotenoids in zucchini cultivars cultivated in Almeria by liquid chromatography.' *Acta Horticulturae*, (939), 183–187.

Kurz, C., et al. 2008. 'HPLC-DAD-MSn characterisation of carotenoids from apricots and pumpkins for the evaluation of fruit product authenticity.' *Food Chemistry*, 110(2), 522–530.

Liu, G., Liang, L., Yu, G., & Li, Q. 2018. 'Pumpkin polysaccharide modifies the gut microbiota during alleviation of type 2 diabetes in rats.' *International Journal of Biological Macromolecules*, 115, 711–717.

Martínez-Valdivieso, D., et al. 2014. 'Application of near-infrared reflectance spectroscopy for predicting carotenoid content in summer squash fruit.' *Computers and Electronics in Agriculture*, 108, 71–79.

Massolo, Juan F., et al. 2019. 'Maturity at harvest and postharvest quality of summer squash.' *Pesquisa Agropecuária Brasileira*, 54, e00133.

Muntean, E., Lazăr, V., & Muntean, N. 2008. 'HPLC - PDA Analysis of carotenoids and chlorophylls from *Cucurbita pepo* var. *giromontina* fruits.' *Bulletin of University of Agricultural Sciences and Veterinary Medicine Cluj-Napoca. Agriculture*, 62.

Murkovic, M., Mülleder, U., & Neunteufl, H. 2002. 'Carotenoid content in different varieties of pumpkins.' *Journal of Food Composition and Analysis*, 15(6), 633–638.

Obrero, Á., et al. 2013. 'Carotenogenic gene expression and carotenoid accumulation in three varieties of *cucurbita pepo* during fruit development.' *Journal of Agricultural and Food Chemistry*, 61(26), 6393–6403.

Oloyede, F. M., Agbaje, G. O., Obuotor, E. M., & Obisesan, I. O. 2012. 'Nutritional and antioxidant profiles of pumpkin (*Cucurbita pepo* Linn.) immature and mature fruits as influenced by NPK fertilizer.' *Food Chemistry*, 135(2), 460–463.

Pezdirc, K., et al. 2016. 'Consuming high-carotenoid fruit and vegetables influences skin yellowness and plasma carotenoids in young women: A single-blind randomized crossover trial.' *Journal of the Academy of Nutrition and Dietetics*, 116(8), 1257–1265.

Provesi, J. G., & Amante, E. R. 2015. 'Carotenoids in pumpkin and impact of processing treatments and storage.' *Processing and Impact on Active Components in Food*, 71–80.

Sharma, Sonu & Ramana Rao, T. V. 2013. 'Nutritional quality characteristics of pumpkin fruit as revealed by its biochemical analysis.' *International Food Research Journal*, 20(5), 2309-2316.

Tarhan, L., Kayali, H.A. & Urek, R.O. 2007. 'In vitro antioxidant properties of *Cucurbita Pepo* L. male and female flowers extracts.' *Plant Foods for Human Nutrition*, 62(2), 49-51.

The legume family
A.S.M. Golam Masum Akond, et al. 2011. 'Anthocyanin, total polyphenols and antioxidant activity of common bean.' *American Journal of Food Technology*, 6, 385-394.

Boschin, G., & Arnoldi, A. 2011. 'Legumes are valuable sources of tocopherols.' *Food Chemistry*, 127(3), 1199–1203.

Fabbri, A. D. T., Schacht, R. W., & Crosby, G. A. 2016. 'Evaluation of resistant starch content of cooked black beans, pinto beans, and chickpeas.' *NFS Journal*, 3, 8–12.

Goławska, S., Kapusta, I., Lukasik, I., & Wójcicka, A. (2008). 'Effect of phenolics on the pea aphid, *Acyrthosiphon pisum* [Harris] population on *Pisum sativum* L.' *Pesticides*, 3-4, 71-77.

Khan, M. K., et al. 2015. 'Phytochemical composition and bioactivities of lupin: a review.' *International Journal of Food Science & Technology*, 50(9), 2004–2012.

Khang, D., Dung, T., Elzaawely, A., & Xuan, T. 2016. 'Phenolic profiles and antioxidant activity of germinated legumes.' *Foods*, 5(4), 27.

Maphosa, Y., & Jideani, V. A. 2017. 'The role of legumes in human nutrition.' *Functional Food - Improve Health through Adequate Food*, Intech, Croatia.

Moriyama, H., et al. 2003. 'Superoxide anion-scavenging activity of anthocyanin pigments.' *Nippon Shokuhin Kagaku Kogaku Kaishi*, 50(11), 499–505.

Rebello, C. J., et al. 2014. 'A review of the nutritional value of legumes and their effects on obesity and its related co-morbidities.' *Obesity Reviews*, 15(5), 392–407.

Rochfort, S., & Panozzo, J. 2007. 'Phytochemicals for health, the role of pulses.' *Journal of Agricultural and Food Chemistry*, 55(20), 7981–7994.

Scher, Caroline, Fenner, Brandelli, Adriano, & Noreña, Caciano Zapata. 2015. 'Yacon inulin leaching during hot water blanching.' *Ciência e Agrotecnologia*, 39(5), 523-529.

Xu, B. J., Yuan, S. H., & Chang, S. K. C. 2007. 'Comparative analyses of phenolic composition, antioxidant capacity, and color of cool season legumes and other selected food legumes.' *Journal of Food Science*, 72(2), S167–S177.

Sweetcorn
Dewanto, V., Wu, X., & Liu, R. H. 2002. 'Processed sweet corn has higher antioxidant activity.' *Journal of Agricultural and Food Chemistry*, 50(17), 4959–4964.

Jing, P., Noriega, V., Schwartz, S. J., & Giusti, M. M. 2007. 'Effects of growing conditions on purple corncob (*Zea mays L.*) anthocyanins.' *Journal of Agricultural and Food Chemistry*, 55(21), 8625–8629.

Khampas, S. & Lertrat, K., Lomthaisong, K. & Suriharn, B. 2013. 'Variability in phytochemicals and antioxidant activity in corn at immaturity and physiological maturity stages.' *International Food Research Journal*, 20(6), 3149-3157.

Siyuan, S., Tong, L., & Liu, R. H. 2018. 'Corn phytochemicals and their health benefits.' *Food Science and Human Wellness*, 7(3), 185-195.

Xiang, N., et al. 2017. 'Effect of light- and dark-germination on the phenolic biosynthesis, phytochemical profiles, and antioxidant activities in sweetcorn sprouts.' *International Journal of Molecular Sciences*, 18(6), 1246.

The potato family
Antonious, G. F. 2014. 'Impact of soil management practices on yield, fruit quality, and antioxidant contents of pepper at four stages of fruit development.' *Journal of Environmental Science and Health*, Part B, 49(10), 769–774.

B.D. Whitaker, J.R. Stommel. 2013. 'Distribution of hydroxycinnamic acids in fruit of commercial eggplant (*Solanum melongena* L.) cultivars.' *Journal of Agricultural and Food Chemistry*, 51, 3448-3454

Barbagallo, R. N., Di Silvestro, I., & Patanè, C. 2012. 'Yield, physicochemical traits, antioxidant pattern, polyphenol oxidase activity and total visual quality of field-grown processing tomato cv. Brigade as affected by water stress in Mediterranean climate.' *Journal of the Science of Food and Agriculture*, 93(6), 1449–1457.

Campos, M. R. S., et al. 2013. 'Polyphenols, ascorbic acid and carotenoids contents and antioxidant properties of habanero pepper (*Capsicum chinense*) fruit.' *Food and Nutrition Sciences*, 4(8), 47–54.

DeWeerdt, S. 2011. 'Food: The omnivore's labyrinth.' *Nature*, 471(7339), S22–S24.

Djouadi, A., Lanez, T., & Boubekri, C. 2016. 'Evaluation of antioxidant activity and polyphenolic contents of two South Algerian eggplants cultivars.' *Journal of Fundamental and Applied Sciences*, 8(2), 223.

Ezekiel, R., Singh, N., Sharma, S., & Kaur, A. 2013. 'Beneficial phytochemicals in potato — a review.' *Food Research International*, 50(2), 487–496.

Gürbüz, N., et al. 2018. 'Health benefits and bioactive compounds of eggplant.' *Food Chemistry*, 268, 602–610.

Hallmann, E. 2012. 'The influence of organic and conventional cultivation systems on the nutritional value and content of bioactive compounds in selected tomato types.' *Journal of the Science of Food and Agriculture*, 92(14), 2840–2848.

Hanson, P. M., et al. 2006. 'Diversity in eggplant (*Solanum melongena*) for superoxide scavenging activity, total phenolics, and ascorbic acid.' *Journal of Food Composition and Analysis*, 19(6-7), 594–600.

Hwang, I. G., et al. 2012. 'Effects of different cooking methods on the antioxidant properties of red pepper (*Capsicum annuum* L.).' *Preventive Nutrition and Food Science*, 17(4), 286–292.

J. Dias. 2012. 'Nutritional quality and health benefits of vegetables: A review,' *Food and Nutrition Sciences*, 3 (10), 1354-1374.

Kaur, C., et al. 2014. 'Evaluating eggplant (Solanum melongena L.) genotypes for bioactive properties: A chemometric approach.' *Food Research International*, 60, 205–211.

Kevers, C., et al. 2007. 'Evolution of antioxidant capacity during storage of selected fruits and vegetables.' *Journal of Agricultural and Food Chemistry*, 55(21), 8596–8603.

Kubota, C., et al. 2006. 'Controlled Environments for Production of Value-added Food Crops with High Phytochemical Concentrations: Lycopene in Tomato as an Example, *HortScience*, 41(3), 522-525.

Loizzo, M. R., et al. 2015. 'Evaluation of chemical profile and antioxidant activity of twenty cultivars from *Capsicum annuum, Capsicum baccatum, Capsicum chacoense* and *Capsicum chinense*: A comparison between fresh and processed peppers.' *LWT - Food Science and Technology*, 64(2), 623–631.

Niño-Medina, G., et al. 2017. 'Structure and content of phenolics in eggplant – a review.' *South African Journal of Botany*, 111, 161–169.

Plazas, M., et al. 2013. 'Breeding for chlorogenic acid content in eggplant: Interest and prospects.' *Notulae Botanicae Horti Agrobotanici Cluj-Napoca*, 41(1), 26.

Raatz, S. K., et al. 2016. 'Resistant starch analysis of commonly consumed potatoes: Content varies by cooking method and service temperature but not by variety.' *Food Chemistry*, 208, 297–300.

Riahi, A., & Hdider, C. 2013. 'Bioactive compounds and antioxidant activity of organically grown tomato cultivars as affected by fertilization.' *Scientia Horticulturae, 151*, 90–96.

Slimestad, R., & Verheul, M. 2009. 'Review of flavonoids and other phenolics from fruits of different tomato (*Lycopersicon esculentum* Mill.) cultivars.' *Journal of the Science of Food and Agriculture*, 89(8), 1255–1270.

Vela-Hinojosa, C., et al. 2019. 'Antioxidant balance and regulation in tomato genotypes of different color.' *Journal of the American Society for Horticultural Science*, 144(1), 45-54.

Zaheer, K., & Akhtar, M. H. 2014. 'Potato production, usage, and nutrition—A review.' *Critical Reviews in Food Science and Nutrition*, 56(5), 711–721.

Herbs
Pérez-Jiménez, J., Neveu, V., Vos, F., & Scalbert, A. 2010. 'Identification of the 100 richest dietary sources of polyphenols.' *European Journal of Clinical Nutrition*, 64(S3), S112–S120.

Dhami, N., & Mishra, A. D. 2015. 'Phytochemical variation: How to resolve the quality controversies of herbal medicinal products?' *Journal of Herbal Medicine*, 5(2), 118–127.

Jarić, S., Mitrović, M., & Pavlović, P. 2015. 'Review of ethnobotanical, phytochemical, and pharmacological study of *Thymus serpyllum* L.' *Evidence-Based Complementary and Alternative Medicine*, 2015, 1–10.

Duda, S. C., et al. 2015. 'Changes in major bioactive compounds with antioxidant activity of *Agastache foeniculum, Lavandula angustifolia, Melissa officinalis* and *Nepeta cataria*: Effect of harvest time and plant species.' *Industrial Crops and Products, 77,* 499–507.

Priecina, L. & Karklina, D. 2014. 'Natural antioxidant changes in fresh and dried spices and vegetables.' *International Journal of Nutrition and Food Engineering, 8 (5),* 492-496.

Opara, E., & Chohan, M. 2014. 'Culinary herbs and spices: their bioactive properties, the contribution of polyphenols and the challenges in deducing their true health benefits.' *International Journal of Molecular Sciences*, 15(10), 19183–19202.

Yi, W., & Wetzstein, H. Y. 2011. 'Effects of drying and extraction conditions on the biochemical activity of selected herbs.' *HortScience, 46(1), 70–73.

Apples
Fang, T., et al. 2017. 'Variation of ascorbic acid concentration in fruits of cultivated and wild apples.' *Food Chemistry*, 225, 132–137.

Gerhauser, C. 2008. 'Cancer chemopreventive potential of apples, apple juice, and apple components.' *Planta Medica*, 74(13), 1608–1624.

Han, M., et al. 2019. 'Phenolic profile, antioxidant activity and anti-proliferative activity of crabapple fruits.' *Horticultural Plant Journal*, 5(4), 155-163.

Hyson, D. A. 2011. 'A comprehensive review of apples and apple components and their relationship to human health.' *Advances in Nutrition*, 2(5), 408–420.

Imeh, U., & Khokhar, S. 2002. 'Distribution of conjugated and free phenols in fruits: antioxidant activity and cultivar variations.' *Journal of Agricultural and Food Chemistry*, 50(22), 6301–6306.

Kahle, K., Kraus, M., & Richling, E. 2005. 'Polyphenol profiles of apple juices.' *Molecular Nutrition & Food Research*, 49(8), 797–806.

Kalinowska, M., et al. 2014. 'Apples: Content of phenolic compounds vs. variety, part of apple and cultivation model, extraction of phenolic compounds, biological properties.' *Plant Physiology and Biochemistry*, 84, 169–188.

Kschonsek, J., et al. 2018. 'Polyphenolic compounds analysis of old and new apple cultivars and contribution of polyphenolic profile to the in vitro antioxidant capacity.' *Antioxidants (Basel, Switzerland)*, 7(1), 20.

Míguez, B., et al. 2016. 'Pectic oligosaccharides and other emerging prebiotics.' *Probiotics and Prebiotics in Human Nutrition and Health*, InTech Open.

Sun, J., Chu, Y.-F., Wu, X., & Liu, R. H. 2002. 'Antioxidant and antiproliferative activities of common fruits.' *Journal of Agricultural and Food Chemistry*, 50(25), 7449–7454.

Tsao, R., et al. 2005. 'Which polyphenolic compounds contribute to the total antioxidant activities of apples?' *Journal of Agricultural and Food Chemistry*, 53(12), 4989–4995.

Weichselbaum, E., et al. 2010. 'Apple polyphenols and cardiovascular disease - a review of the evidence.' *Nutrition Bulletin*, 35(2), 92–101.

Pears
Galvis Sánchez, A. C., Gil-Izquierdo, A., & Gil, M. I. 2003. 'Comparative study of six pear cultivars in terms of their phenolic and vitamin C contents and antioxidant capacity.' *Journal of the Science of Food and Agriculture*, 83(10), 995–1003.

Kevers, C., et al. 2011. 'Influence of cultivar, harvest time, storage conditions, and peeling on the antioxidant capacity and phenolic and ascorbic acid contents of apples and pears.' *Journal of Agricultural and Food Chemistry*, 59(11), 6165–6171.

Kolniak-Ostek, J. 2016. 'Chemical composition and antioxidant capacity of different anatomical parts of pear.' *Food Chemistry*, 203, 491–497.

Li, X., Li, X., Wang, T., & Gao, W. 2016. 'Nutritional composition of pear cultivars.' *Nutritional Composition of Fruit Cultivars*, 573–608.

Makkumrai, W., et al. 2014. 'Effect of ethylene and temperature conditioning on sensory attributes and chemical composition of 'Bartlett' pears.' *Postharvest Biology and Technology*, 97, 44–61.

Reiland, H., & Slavin, J. 2015. 'Systematic review of pears and health.' *Nutrition Today*, 50(6), 301–305.

Peaches
Asami, D. K., Hong, Y.-J., Barrett, D. M., & Mitchell, A. E. 2003. 'Processing-induced changes in total phenolics and procyanidins in clingstone peaches.' *Journal of the Science of Food and Agriculture*, 83(1), 56–63.

Buendía, B., et al. 2008. 'Effect of regulated deficit irrigation and crop load on the antioxidant compounds of peaches.' *Journal of Agricultural and Food Chemistry*, 56(10), 3601–3608.

Gil, M. I., et al. 2002. 'Antioxidant capacities, phenolic compounds, carotenoids, and vitamin C contents of nectarine, peach, and plum cultivars from California.' *Journal of Agricultural and Food Chemistry, 50(17), 4976–4982*.

Pliakoni, E. D., & Nanos, G. D. 2010. 'Deficit irrigation and reflective mulch effects on peach and nectarine fruit quality and storage ability.' *Acta Horticulturae*, (877), 215–222.

Puerta-Gomez, A. F., & Cisneros-Zevallos, L. 2011. 'Postharvest studies beyond fresh market eating quality: Phytochemical antioxidant changes in peach and plum fruit during ripening and advanced senescence.' *Postharvest biology and technology*, 60, 220-224.

Remorini, D., et al. 2008. 'Effect of rootstocks and harvesting time on the nutritional quality of peel and flesh of peaches fruits.' *Food Chemistry*, 110(2), 361–367.

Scattino, C., et al. 2014. 'Post-harvest UV-B irradiation induces changes of phenol contents and corresponding biosynthetic gene expression in peaches and nectarines.' *Food Chemistry*, 163, 51–60.

Tsantili, E., Shin, Y., Nock, J. F., & Watkins, C. B. 2010. 'Antioxidant concentrations during chilling injury development in peaches.' *Postharvest Biology and Technology*, 57(1), 27–34.

Vizzotto, M., et al. 2014. 'Polyphenols of selected peach and plum genotypes reduce cell viability and inhibit proliferation of breast cancer cells while not affecting normal cells.' *Food Chemistry*, 164, 363–370.

Berries
Beekwilder, J., et al. 2005. 'Identification and dietary relevance of antioxidants from raspberry.' *BioFactors, 23*(4), 197–205.

Giovanelli, G., & Buratti, S. 2009. 'Comparison of polyphenolic composition and antioxidant activity of wild Italian blueberries and some cultivated varieties.' *Food Chemistry*, 112(4), 903–908.

Jaakola, L., et al. 2017. 'Influence of light and temperature conditions on anthocyanin accumulation in *Vaccinium* spp. berries.' *Acta Horticulturae*, (1180), 321–326.

Jeong, J.-C. et al. 2015. 'Growing environment influence the anthocyanin content in purple- and red-fleshed potatoes during tuber development.' *Korean Journal of Crop Science, 60(2), 231-238*.

Jezek, M., Zörb, C., Merkt, N., & Geilfus, C.-M. 2018. 'Anthocyanin management in fruits by fertilization.' *Journal of Agricultural and Food Chemistry*, 66(4), 753–764.

Kaume, L., Howard, L. R., & Devareddy, L. 2011. 'The blackberry fruit: a review on its composition and chemistry, metabolism and bioavailability, and health benefits.' *Journal of Agricultural and Food Chemistry*, 60(23), 5716–5727.

Kraft B.T.F., et al. 2008. 'Phytochemical composition and metabolic performance-enhancing activity of dietary berries traditionally used by native north Americans.' *Journal of Agriculture and Food Chemistry, 56, 654–660*

Mikulic-Petkovsek, M., et al. 2012. 'HPLC-MSn identification and quantification of flavonol glycosides in 28 wild and cultivated berry species.' *Food Chemistry*, 135(4), 2138–2146.

Pérez-Jiménez, J., Neveu, V., Vos, F., & Scalbert, A. 2010. 'Identification of the 100 richest dietary sources of polyphenols: an application of the Phenol-Explorer database.' *European Journal of Clinical Nutrition*, 64(S3), S112–S120.

Wang, Y., et al. 2016. 'Comparison of polyphenol, anthocyanin and antioxidant capacity in four varieties of *Lonicera caerulea* berry extracts.' *Food Chemistry*, 197, 522–529.

Plums
Arjmandi, B. H., et al. 2002. 'Dried plums improve indices of bone formation in postmenopausal women.' *Journal of Women's Health & Gender-Based Medicine*, 11(1), 61–68.

Fanning, K., et al. 2013. 'Increasing anthocyanin content in Queen Garnet plum and correlations with in-field measures.' *Acta Horticulturae*, (985), 97–104.

Igwe, E. O., & Charlton, K. E. 2016. 'A systematic review on the health effects of plums (*Prunus domestica* and *Prunus salicina*).' *Phytotherapy Research*, 30(5), 701–731.

Madrau, M. A., et al. 2010. 'Contribution of melanoidins to the antioxidant activity of prunes.' *Journal of Food Quality*, 33, 155–170.

Melgarejo, P., et al. 2012. 'Chemical, functional and quality properties of Japanese plum (Prunus salicina Lindl.) as affected by mulching.' *Scientia Horticulturae*, 134, 114–120.

Rop, O., et al. 2009. 'Antioxidant activity and selected nutritional values of plums typical of the White Carpathian Mountains.' *Scientia Horticulturae*, 122(4), 545–549.

Figs
Bey, M. B., & Louaileche, H. 2015. 'A comparative study of phytochemical profile and in vitro antioxidant activities of dark and light dried fig (*Ficus carica* L.) varieties.' *The Journal of Phytopharmacology*, 4(1), 41-48.

Harzallah, A., et al. 2016. 'Phytochemical content and antioxidant activity of different fruit parts juices of three fig varieties grown in Tunisia.' *Industrial Crops and Products*, 83, 255–267.

Kamiloglu, S., & Capanoglu, E. 2014. 'Polyphenol content in figs (*Ficus carica* L.): Effect of sun-drying.' *International Journal of Food Properties*, 18(3), 521–535.

Palmeira, L., et al. 2019. 'Nutritional, chemical and bioactive profiles of different parts of a Portuguese common fig (*Ficus carica* L.) variety.' *Food Research International*, 126, 108572.

Veberic, R., Colaric, M., & Stampar, F. 2008. 'Phenolic acids and flavonoids of fig fruit (*Ficus carica* L.) in the northern Mediterranean region.' *Food Chemistry*, 106(1), 153–157.

Index

Page numbers in **bold** indicate a main entry and those in *italics* an illustration, caption or shaded box.

Photography credits

All photography: Marianne Majerus
(mariannemajerus.com) except:

p.29 David Richter
Shutterstock: p.37 no 2, Tami Freed;
p.109 no.2 ThaiThu;
p.111 no.2 Ivan Marjanovic;
p.119 no. 1 arjma; p.121 Picmin;
p.160 (Chia) The natures

Acknowledgments

Author's acknowledgments

First and foremost, thank you to my partner David for being so wonderful and supportive throughout the entire duration of me writing this book. I literally could not have done it without you. Thank you also for meticulously drawing the illustrations for the book, they are beautiful. Thank you Frank and Fern for entertaining Daddy.

Thank you to our wonderful employers, for inspiring the idea and allowing me to experiment so extensively with the edible garden.

Thank you to Marianne for all your skill and professionalism, working long hours to get the best images of the garden, and kindly tolerating the frequent baby-related interruptions. It's been great fun creating the book together and I've learnt so much from you. Thank you also to your husband Robert for tolerating all our incursions into his free time, and for providing impromptu childcare services.

My heartfelt thanks to all the editorial team from Frances Lincoln: Helen Griffin, Zia Allaway, Rachel Cross and Bella Skertchly. Thank you for putting your trust in me to write the book as an untested writer, for helping me to make the book more practical and accessible to the reader, and for going to such great lengths to design the book so beautifully. It really has been an incredible team effort.

Thank you to Dr Caroline Le Roy, Research Associate at King's College London, who is an expert in the interactions between diet and the gut microbiota and how this affects our metabolism. Thanks very much for our conversations on the subject, reviewing my research, checking that it is factually correct, and suggesting very interesting additional references. It is a real challenge to interpret the scientific literature to give practical gardening advice and you have really given me confidence in my arguments.

Many thanks to Charles Dowding, expert organic grower and leading authority on no dig gardening, for taking the time to read a draft of the book and provide very helpful constructive criticism and advice.

Thank you very much to my key fermentation recipe 'tasters' Agi and Cristina for gamely trying all the concoctions I've come up with and giving me your honest opinions. You've really helped me to hone the recipes.

I'm indebted to the scientific community for their fascinating research which, despite reading innumerable papers, I feel I have barely scratched the surface of exploring.

Thank you to the social media community on Instagram. You've been a real source of inspiration. Your comments and questions have really helped me focus.

Thank you to Julia Leakey and Ann Hutchinson at Crocus for kindly supplying me with essential pots for my projects.

Last but not least, thank you to all my friends and family who've given me so much encouragement and support and have helped to make this book a reality.

For further updates on this fascinating subject, please visit my Instagram @guthealthgardener.

Photographer's acknowledgments

I would like to thank Beth for being such a pleasure to work with, and David, Frank and Fern for being the back-up team and providing the entertainment. Thanks also to my husband Robert, as well as Bennet and Martin, for their invaluable help, and the team at Frances Lincoln for their vision and dedication in making this project a reality.

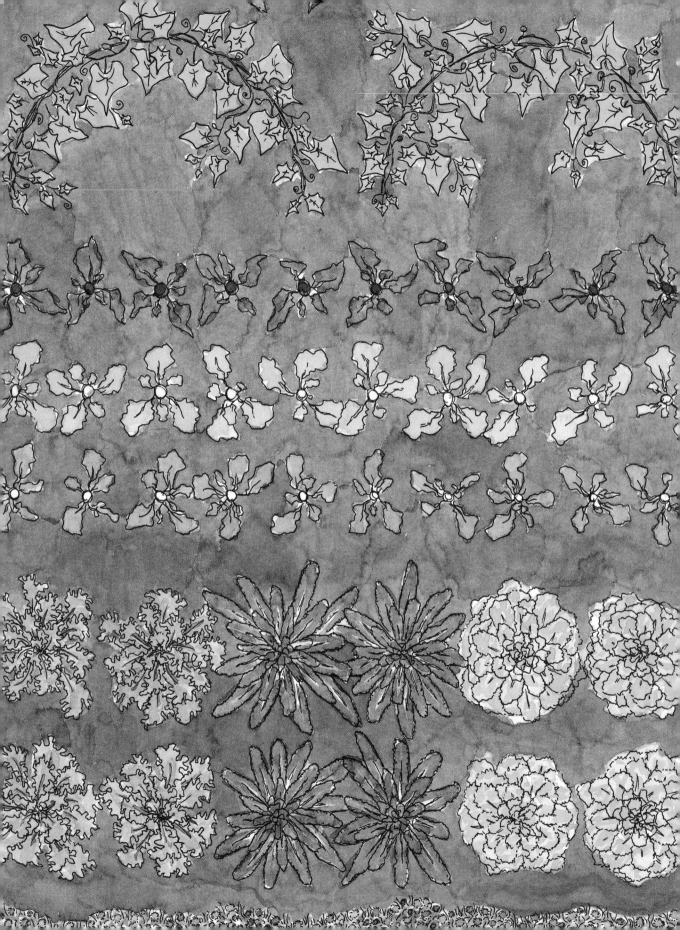